# how to

# stay sane

# on the

# baby

# making

# train

# how to stay sane on the baby making train

BERNADETTE ANDREWS

the kind press

Cover design: Mila Graphic Artist
Internal design by Nicola Matthews, Nikki Jane Design
Edited by Georgia Gordan
Author photo credit: Jade Stewart

Cataloguing-in-Publication entry is available from the National Library Australia.

NATIONAL
LIBRARY
OF AUSTRALIA

ISBN: 978-0-6451392-6-6
ISBN: 978-0-6451392-5-9 (ebook)

*This book is dedicated to my husband, Quentin,*

*who is the best thing in my life.*

*And to all my readers, please know that you are*

*not alone on this journey.*

**The baby making train:** You get on and it speeds up while you are all wide eyed and excited with anticipation, but the excitement gradually slows down when you don't pick up any new bundles of joy along the journey. Sometimes the train is full and bustling with activity, other times it is all empty and alone, sitting and waiting. There are times you are happy to jump on, other times you can't wait to get off and back to normal. Sometimes it's really expensive, other times you score a free ticket. Sometimes the train driver and attendants are cheery and helpful, other times it's their last shift on a long day. When and where will this train ride stop while on this unknown journey?

# Contents

# Introduction

*Life is 10% what happens to you*
*and 90% how you react to it.*
—Charles R Swindoll

With one in six couples experiencing infertility, why is it that no one talks about it openly? Why do so many couples suffer in silence? Why do we feel like a failure when we don't conceive on cue?

When you think about the reproductive process, it's kind of a miracle that anyone falls pregnant and gives birth to a healthy baby in the first place, right? There are so many obstacles that come to mind, such as finding a partner, age, general health, work/money/lifestyle stresses, the timing of the egg release, quality of the egg and sperm, clear tubes, a good-looking uterus to implant in, morning sickness, no drinking alcohol, no drugs, no smoking, no eating soft cheese, processed meats or shellfish, risk of miscarriage in any trimester, a healthy fetus growing for nine months, vaginal delivery or caesarean surgery … and after all that, fingers crossed that the baby comes out screaming and that the mother and father are alive. Wow, I'm actually surprised that we are even born after all that we have to go through to get here.

Therefore, with the chances of even falling pregnant lean to start with, why do we feel so ashamed of not being able to? Why do we feel we have to suffer in silence and that we don't have a purpose in life if we want children but can't have them? And why do we lose ourselves and our sense of purpose on the baby-making train ride when suddenly the heartfelt joy of starting a family gets taken over by doctors, numbers, cold white clinics, crazy medical bills, early morning appointments before work, and crossing all fingers and toes with the hope that this time it will work?

There are many books and websites out there on how to get pregnant, what to eat, what to do, how long for, etc. There are websites on who is the best doctor, clinic, alternative therapist. How do we not lose ourselves on this crazy baby-making train ride—our sense of self, spirit, lightness, freedom, joy and play—when every day we are trying to obtain something that we can't? And not for lack of trying.

It hasn't been very long since the traditional role of a woman was to get married young and have children. Ever since men were the hunters and women the home-making gatherers. Married, childless women throughout history were treated terribly even though in a percentage of the couples it was actually the male who medically couldn't have children. The blame was only ever put on the women with the term "barren" used when referring to them. Such a harsh word, meaning incapable of producing offspring.

However, now in a post-feminist world there are many roles for women other than mother. Women can now have careers, travel, be members of parliament, join the defence force, be an astronaut, even be the prime minister or president of a country. There are so many more options now than ever before.

I have been on and off the baby making train since I was twenty-four years old and I am now forty. The struggle for me was mostly in silent moments, especially in the early days—questioning myself with *Why me? Everyone else is pregnant, why can't I be?*

In my twenties to early thirties, I wasn't completely happy within myself as I thought my only purpose in this world was to be a mother, therefore I thought that a baby would make me happy, make me whole.

However, the struggle in silence was real. I looked happy on the outside, but inside it was all I ever thought about … my lack of a baby. I was living for a future state: *When I have a baby I will be happy, when I have a baby I will have my purpose in life, when I have a baby I will be able to join the mothers club.* It was like I was missing out when everyone else was blissfully happy.

If you are reading this book, you are most likely on your own journey of the baby making train. The purpose of this book is to inspire and encourage you to not lose your sense of self on the baby making train. That you as a person are already whole and complete regardless of a baby. You will be able to love and nurture yourself more. You will know what to say to *that* question (you know the one), and you will feel confident

# About me

Throughout my journey on the baby-making train, I have at times been one hundred per cent committed to falling pregnant, like a dog chasing a bone, other times I have been off the train completely, going on overseas holidays, learning new things, eating and drinking all the things you're probably not supposed to when you are on the baby making train.

I excitedly walked up to the Baby Making Platform when I was twenty-four, ready and willing for this next adventurous ride. However, the train must have been delayed as I patiently waited and waited but it never turned up, not even once.

From the age of twenty-seven to thirty-one I was full steam ahead on the assisted baby making train. On the train ride with me were doctors, naturopaths, Chinese medicine acupuncturists, IVF doctors and nurses.

I fell off the train from about thirty-two to thirty-four when the train fully derailed by going completely off course without a driver; the signals malfunctioned and we were crashing around in the dark trying to course correct.

When I turned thirty-five our baby making train went into

the service department to get fixed. And by the time I was thirty-six it was sparkling, with all-new shining parts, however by the end of that year a sudden storm came over without warning and the train just stayed parked with a *Not in service* sign in the front window—where it still currently sits.

When on the baby making train, I have struggled with the *Why is everyone else falling pregnant but me?* question. Why can't I at least have one baby when others are falling pregnant with their third, fourth surprises? Why is it so hard? Why is it so expensive when others get drunk and fall pregnant on a one-night stand? It seemed that everyone else was easily falling pregnant, but I was having such a hard time trying to get pregnant … there was no easy "falling" for me.

When I was on the baby making train in the "one hundred per cent committed to getting pregnant" zone, I keep it mostly to myself: only a few close family and friends knew. I felt like there was something wrong with me. I saw pregnant bellies everywhere I went. Some friends and family gave me their used baby clothes and items, which sat in my spare room (the room which had been waiting for so long to be turned into a nursery for years) before I eventually took it all to the op shop.

Everything revolved around trying to get pregnant. If we went on holidays, would I be in the middle of an IVF treatment where I had to take daily timed injections, medication, Chinese herbs, etc.? With work, if I was in my busiest time of the year, would I be stressed during treatment and therefore paying all this money for IVF for nothing because I had work stress? If I was in the two-week wait period after an embryo transfer, I had to plan it so that I didn't have any big work meetings, a family function or a sporting weekend, and I wasn't allowed to exercise during that resting time.

I really lost my sense of self; who was I if I didn't have children? Was life worth living if I wasn't a mother? Was anyone else out there going through what I was going through? Because I didn't really know anyone else who was early on.

I always knew what day of my monthly cycle I was on without looking at my diary. When we travelled I thought of my struggle to get pregnant. If we went for a nice drive along a beautiful coastline, I would be thinking of my lack of a baby. Sometimes while watching a movie, concert or show I would have thoughts of *Why am I not pregnant?* It seriously invaded every waking moment.

Growing up the youngest of five children in a Catholic family, I was always playing with dolls with my sisters. Whether it be Barbie dolls, Cabbage Patch Kids or ugly lifelike infant dolls ... even our pet cats would be dressed up in dolls clothes and wheeled around in our dolls pram, much to their distaste.

We also had heaps of space to roam around as we grew up on a farm and there was always so much to explore. However, every Sunday morning without fail we went to church.

My parents were away one weekend, leaving my eldest brother in charge, and instead of the cliché of throwing a party, we wagged church and decided to sleep in, such rebels.

But like always, Mum found out. So the next weekend we had to go to confession before church, which is where you go into a room and tell the priest what your sins are, and he will tell you how many Hail Marys you must say in your prayers.

Well, I went into confession and told the priest that I had not sinned at all. He totally didn't believe me but I was good to go with three Hail Mary prayers.

In school I remember we learnt about family structures, and when looking at mine I had the perfect nuclear family ... Mum and Dad and full-blooded brothers and sisters. How perfect were we. However, when I was fifteen my father got sick and passed away five months later. He was only fifty-six years old, leaving my mum a widow at only forty-six. How very young this sounds to me now.

After Dad passed away it was suddenly just Mum and me at home, as my siblings had all finished school and left home to work or study. Hang on a sec—where did my perfect nuclear family go?

Dad had really been the head of our family and worked six to seven days a week on the farm and in various businesses. So it was hard to see a very fit and active person suddenly be in a wheelchair and lying in a hospital bed weak and vulnerable.

My mum was suddenly forced to handle the running of the household as well as keep an eye on my four siblings, as they were all living in different towns and cities at the time and I was in high school—everyone was all over the place. It was a huge adjustment for me, and I had to grow up quickly.

My dad really encouraged my sisters and me to study, learn and get careers, so that we wouldn't have to rely on a man or work in the very hard conditions of farm life. So when I finished high school I went on to study for a diploma in business travel.

However, when I selected my preferences in grade 12 I didn't really know what the travel part meant, I just saw the word "business", which is what I had wanted to study. Little did I know that the "travel" part of the course name actually meant working in the travel industry. I had never even been on a plane, let alone known that there was an industry such as travel.

Well funny how things work out, as I ended up working in corporate travel for the next twenty years.

I met my husband when I was eighteen. He had just turned twenty-one and recently finished university. My flatmate had just started dating a guy (her husband now too) and she had met my husband at his twenty-first birthday party and thought he would be perfect for me. Only problem was that he was dating someone else at the time. However, about a week or so later he was single and my flatmate set up a blind double date. I was attracted to him straight away as he was nice and tall (all the other boys in high school were shorter than me). And I loved that he smiled a lot when he was talking, as it showed him to be a lighthearted, fun person … not too serious.

We got married when I was twenty-two. It sounds so young now but at the time I was ready to settle down. And a few close friends were getting married as well. And the natural next step was to buy our first home, which we did when I was twenty-four.

We didn't have much furniture in our home, our dining table was a plastic green outdoor setting and our curtains were sheets pinned to the walls. However, even though we were saving up to finish off our little home, I thought *Ok, let's have a baby*. I worked in the city and commuted an hour and a half each way to work and because I was unhappy with my long workdays, I thought that I would have a baby so that I could stay at home ... well it beats going to work and sitting on a train for hours, so I thought!

Well, guess what? After six months I hadn't fallen pregnant.

Our baby-making train ride to date has involved many GP visits, numerous referrals to IVF specialists, blood doctor specialists, consultations with naturopaths face to face, online or via Zoom, many blood tests (to my distaste), peeing into cups, taking basal body temperatures daily, cooking up Chinese herbs that taste like dirt, taking a million supplements and homeopathic remedies, getting jabbed in the belly with IVF injections, experiencing numerous scans in lovely positions, cooking up a storm when following fertility eating plans, taking time off work to go to various appointments, and talking to close friends and family about the next thing we were going to try.

I have read so many books on the subject of getting pregnant and researched different diets and alternative therapies. I've rearranged furniture, hoping that the feng shui will bring a baby to us. I even bought from a Balinese shop three carved wooden elephants that promised to bring babies if placed in the bedroom; after about six years of dusting them I took them to the op shop.

However, with age there comes wisdom and knowing yourself more. In my early thirties I became more confident within myself, and I could talk a little more about my struggle on the baby making train. I even took myself to a few Saturday morning IVF group coffee and chats. Now I have just embraced forty and after doing a lot of inner work on myself, I am in the best place I have ever been. The future is bright, many adventures await in life. We have so many exciting opportunities available to us, we just need to keep our hearts open to life.

In the following chapters I will share my tips—the good, the bad and all the funny stuff in between—for ultimately staying sane on the baby making train.

# 1

# Why me?

Why is everyone else pregnant and showing off their growing bellies, wearing new and funky maternity clothes, shopping for cute nursery furniture, and endlessly talking about pregnancy and baby names, and not me?

All I see are pregnancy bellies everywhere and the mums-to-be always seem so happy and excited. Even their husbands seem overly happy, like they have joined this amazing new world. I want in.

Oh, but you actually have to fall pregnant and give birth to a baby to join this amazing new world that the majority of the population are in? And is it only me who cannot join in on the fun? Why can't I fall pregnant and have that same pregnancy glow, new clothes, baby showers, baby gifts, new cars, fancy prams that look like they can move on Mars, all the new baby gadgets in the world, pregnancy apps and babymoons? Why can't I go to baby expos or do pregnancy yoga, birthing classes or pregnancy photo shoots with me walking through a beautiful garden with just a white cloth draped for clothing and a hint of pregnancy belly showing as my husband walks slowly beside me, gazing at the belly in awe?

Why is it that everywhere I go I see pregnancy bellies and newborn babies? Just popping down to the shop to pick up milk ... *bang*: pregnancy belly. Just going out to dinner ... *bang*: pregnancy belly. Standing in line at the post office ... *bang*: pregnancy belly. Heading to my fave coffee shop to pick up a latte ... *bang*: a whole table of new mothers with flashy prams, sitting in their activewear and cradling cute newborn babies.

It just feels like pregnancy bellies and babies are everywhere!

It doesn't help that I live in a new suburb that is purpose built for young families. Childcare centres, schools, playgrounds, sporting ovals, bike tracks, jumping gyms, princess parlours, farm petting zoos, etc. are everywhere. It's like the town planners want everyone to procreate.

I like to think that I don't take life too seriously. Cracking a joke and making people laugh is what I'm all about. And I'm usually a very positive person and like to laugh at everything, including myself. However, suffering from infertility has been the one thing in my life that has really challenged my inner sense of joy. At times it has felt like a silent disease. On the outside everything seemed fine but on the inside everything was not.

People would announce their pregnancies and I would congratulate them with joy, asking all the right questions: *How far along? What month are you due? How are you feeling?* And as each of their trimesters went by I would continue with the polite questions: *How is the nursery shopping going? Do you know what sex the baby is? How long are you taking off work?* etc. I even organised the baby showers and would smile, play the silly "sniff the nappy" games and look interested. But inside I felt flattened and deflated, like my usual joke-telling self was about to flip her lid, make a scene and shout from the rooftop *WHY ME!*

I remember one incredibly challenging weekend for me was when my best friend and my sister called me within twenty-four hours of each other to tell me that they were pregnant. Both were surprises and due around the same time. They knew of my struggles and both calls were made from love for me, as they wanted to let me know early on, which I appreciated. However, it was a hard weekend for me to stay positive. It was like a double-edged sword; I was happy for them but felt gutted inside. These were *my* people to share my struggles with and now they were both unexpectedly pregnant—and at the same time. Why them and not me? My sister even said to me that it was supposed to be my turn.

But you have to keep smiling.

And then of course I would go to work and try to stay positive. Put on a smile and walk into the office.

Work and laughing would sometimes help me forget about my *Why me?* woes. My lovely lunch room group really helped with this.

I used to sit with a group of girls, all were different ages and had different jobs around the office. We somehow always seemed to get onto the funniest topics—half the time having no idea how we got onto a particular subject—such as the meaning of the song 'Turning Japanese'. There would be times that we were in tears from laughing so much.

One day one of the girls was saying that twice she went off the pill and just had to *look* at her husband and bang: she was pregnant. She said that she really felt for people who struggle to fall pregnant. And I just sat across the table not saying anything. What would I have said? *Um, yes, well I've been trying to get pregnant for years, done everything including the big one, IVF, and still no baby.* Sometimes it was just easier to carry along, as I didn't want to be a downer on our quick and usually funny lunch breaks. But in my head, I wanted to scream out that it isn't a competition of who falls pregnant the easiest.

And then, another one of the girls who was planning her big wedding had paid for the dress and the reception was all organised, and yes she fell pregnant before the wedding and had to completely change all the wedding plans, etc.

Plus, another girl had finished having her family years ago, was on the pill and everything, but still fell pregnant.

And yet another girl had finished her family, with the husband having had a vasectomy, and she fell pregnant … with twins. WTF!

There has been so many moments of hearing about surprise pregnancies. So many thoughts in my head about why them when they didn't even want it, and not me, who desperately wanted it?

However, there is that saying, *When life gives you lemons, make lemonade.* Everyone on this planet has their own problems, struggles and challenges. There are so many stories of people going through extreme hardship every day. Therefore, instead of looking on the dark and negative side of everything, I think it's best to try and focus on the positive side.

Yes, you will have your *Why me?* times and that is ok to feel that. However, once you have felt that frustration and sadness, try to focus on some more positive thoughts. Such as the fact that you are alive, you are breathing, and if you live in Australia like me, you live in a beautiful country where you are free to walk down the street without getting hit by a suicide bomb. You have the freedom to vote, study at university, run a big corporate company, be a surgeon or pilot, even a politician. These opportunities have only been available to women up until recently.

It is so easy to get sucked into a negative mindset. And it is ok to feel this, but know that it is only for a time as it too shall pass.

For me, instead of just seeing and focusing on everyone else happily pregnant, when I turned my attention back to myself and went within and dug deep there was always a feeling of hope. I definitely had to really dig sometimes, but it was there. That hopeful feeling that next month it could be me unexpectedly finding out that I am pregnant. To do this you need to stop comparing yourself to others, take time out from all the noise, sit with yourself and visualise your own story of happily finding out you're pregnant.

Sometimes the best way to get yourself out of the *Why me?* woes and focusing on your own lack is to redirect that energy to others in need. My husband and I started sponsoring a child through World Vision; he was from Mongolia and we would receive photos of his family standing outside of their home.

Now, this home was definitely not like the houses we are used to, it was pretty much a hut. It felt good to be giving a little to help a child who was really in need. And it helped me get out of that lack mentality and see the bigger picture. So, if I wasn't able to have my own baby right now, at least I could help a child in need and that felt good.

All the stories I have heard and read about people who have gone through and recovered from a major illness—including the big ones such as cancer—all say that they are not the same person they used to be before the diagnosis. That now they stop to smell the roses, they are completely present in a face-to-face conversation instead of looking at their phone, and they celebrate each and every day just for the simple fact that they get to see another day.

Now I'm not suggesting that being on the baby making train is the same as a major illness, however, going through the silent struggles of infertility can have a silver lining. For me, it has strengthened my character. I know that I can handle anything life throws at me. And yes, I've been through many other non-baby-making challenges and I can deal with them without falling into a heap.

It has also strengthened my inner self; I understand myself more as I've had more time to focus on my own inner work. It has also strengthened my relationship with my husband as it is just the two of us and we highly value our time together.

You may not realise it at the time when you are going through it, but when you get knocked down by negative pregnancy tests, a cancelled IVF cycle with no eggs, the blood tests and operations you've nothing to show for apart from medical bills, these setbacks increase your inner strength for any future challenges life may throw at you. This inner power makes you get back up, put one foot in front of the other, take one day at a time and get yourself back out there. This person is a true warrior and that is what you are.

And also, as silly as this may sound—just start smiling more! Smile at yourself in the mirror first thing in the morning, smile when you walk into your workplace, smile when you are out walking the dog, smile to the checkout person. It is amazing that something so simple and free can make you feel so much better. And it is contagious.

It does feel silly to smile when you are feeling sad, but it really helps get you out of the *Why me?* woes. Give it a go, you will instantly feel better.

# staying sane tips

1. *Focus on the good in your life, focus on the amazing surroundings you live in.*

2. *Dig deep within yourself and know that there is always hope for your own pregnancy.*

3. *Redirect your lack-of-a-baby mindset by helping others. Sponsor a child in need.*

4. *As cliché as it sounds, look on the bright side of life. You will feel so much better for it.*

5. *Setbacks and life challenges strengthen your character and your inner self. They strengthen your relationship with yourself and also your life partner. This inner strength will help you overcome anything life may throw at you.*

6. *Put yourself out there and smile. The simple art of smiling at a stranger can be contagious and it will make you feel great!*

# 2

# Please let me join the mothers group

*True belonging is a spiritual practice and it's about the ability to find sacredness in both being a part of something but also the courage to stand alone.*
— Brené Brown

When you are a young child, you don't think much about the future or your life purpose or belonging or legacy. You see your parents, brothers and sisters, schoolteachers, friends, etc. all following a similar path: Go to school, play sport, receive Christmas presents, get cake on your birthday, study, date, start a career, get married, buy a house, have a family, then raise the children to go to school, play sports, give Christmas presents, bake a cake on birthdays, get married, buy a house, have a family. It is a normal pattern that usually ensures belonging and it has been happening for centuries.

Most of us are brought up to believe that our life purpose is to follow this same pattern. When you grow up and meet your life partner, you have and raise a child of your own with similar values to yourself. And so on this pattern repeats on autopilot in the hope that it ensures a sense of belonging or being a part of something bigger than ourselves.

However, this very generalised pattern does not always go to plan. Whether it's wanted or not. If this is your life plan but you fail the step that says you need to have a child and raise that child, then what is your life purpose, legacy and belonging? What pattern do you follow, and has anyone else out there also carved a different pattern, and are they doing ok?

Growing up I never thought I was out of the norm, and I certainly didn't give much thought to my life purpose, legacy and belonging when I was younger. It was just a given that when I grew up and got married I would have a family. That's what my mum did, all my aunties and uncles. Even my uncle and aunty, who didn't have biological children, still had children by adopting. And when my eldest sister got married, she had a baby straight away, even though she had a career as well—she let that go to be a full-time mother.

Hence, when we bought our first home after a couple of years of marriage, we assumed that next would be a baby. We never really talked about children before we got engaged or married as it was just a given that we too would join in on this normal pattern.

A few close friends were having babies around the time that we got married, but I was in no rush as I was only twenty-two. I enjoyed cuddling my friends' new babies, but I also enjoyed handing them back. A couple of years later when I did want a baby of my own, there were probably two reasons for this, and neither was out of love for generally wanting to raise a child.

The first reason was timing: everyone else was starting a family and since we had just bought our first home we thought it was time. The second was probably because I desperately wanted to belong somewhere.

Before I got married, I shared a house with a close group of friends and we would spend every weeknight and weekend pretty much together. Even after I got married, we would still hang out heaps. However, around the time we bought our first home, they moved interstate. So I lost that close friendship group, which was sad because we had been hanging out since we were teenagers.

And I was also very restricted with time to make new friends due to working in the city. Many nights the train didn't get back until late and it was often delayed. I also worked a few Saturdays. Thankfully I did go out on Friday nights with my work friends in the city, which was always heaps of fun, but our homes were all on completely different sides of the city, making it hard to hang out weekends.

There was no time for me to go out after work in the area that I lived to play sport or do something social as the main town from our house was yet another half-hour drive away. And with having to get up early the next day, it was just too much.

Because my husband worked close to home, he was the one getting home early, cooking dinners, watering the garden, playing with our dog and doing the grocery shopping. Whereas I was the one getting home late, eating dinner, showering and going to bed—to do it all over again the next day. This felt really strange to me as it was a role reversal of what I had experienced growing up. Usually, the male was the one getting home late and having their dinner cooked, with the female doing the cooking and grocery shopping.

I felt like I was not fully connected to that home as the restrictions around its location to my work resulted in me feeling lost and like I was trying to carve a new pattern, but I didn't know what that pattern was supposed to look like.

So to help with these feelings of disconnection I thought I should have a baby. This way I could stay home and look after the baby, and there would be no more long train trips to work. I could also meet other new mums in my local area and get a friendship circle where I lived. It was that sense of belonging in my local community I was after. Problem solved!

Well, so I thought.

These are probably not the best reasons to have a baby, but when I was younger I didn't know what I know now and I definitely didn't question anything outside of the status quo.

During those first six months or so of trying for a baby I was kind of secretly excited, but looking back now I was very young and naive. I was only twenty-four years old and I hadn't done any crazy big adventures, such as doing a gap year or working overseas in the UK, as a few of my work friends had done. I was the sensible one who got engaged at twenty-one, married at twenty-two and bought a house at twenty-four.

But at the time I thought that having a baby would sort out my insecurities.

I used to go to the library to get books to read on the long and boring train ride (did I mention the delays?), and they were mostly historical romance novels. Just novels to get enthralled by and pass the time travelling to and from work. Well, at the library they also had the latest copies of mother and baby magazines. I didn't even know that there were such magazines. So I borrowed a few one day and snuck them into the house and put them under my bed as I felt kind of embarrassed for reading them when I wasn't even pregnant. I then would put one in my big handbag and read it on the train, but again I would hide it inside a trashy celebrity magazine so that no one noticed what I was reading.

As the six months turned into twelve months, I just kept feeling sad and like I didn't belong anywhere. Because I was so young I didn't even understand these feelings, I didn't read self-help books or listen to motivation podcasts, or do yoga and meditation as I currently do (being much more common now). There wasn't much information on the topic of self-care and acceptance, it wasn't widely present in the media as it is now. So on I carried in my own world, keeping my feelings to myself.

When I was twenty-five, after we had been trying for a baby for over a year, we went on a holiday to Western Australia. The travel company I worked for ran these tours and as an employee I could do a tour for free, just had to pay for the hubby. So I thought we may as well go do something fun.

We did a three-week camping coach tour from Darwin to Perth. We had such an amazing time as we were with a really fantastic group of people, young backpackers travelling the world. Everything was just about travelling and exploring new places. There was no mobile phone coverage, no internet, no

TV—it was the best holiday to fully disconnect. I went on the pill for that time and totally didn't think about babies or trying to get pregnant. I was just myself again, happy, exploring and being surrounded by interesting people. This holiday started our love of travel.

The next year went by and we had relatives staying with us from interstate. They are very traditional people who believe in going to church every Sunday and having a family as soon as you marry young.

On this particular visit it was a weeknight and when I finally got home from work after the long train trip, I was asked at the dinner table when I was going to have a baby and they read the expression on my face as: *We are trying, but nothing has happened yet.* I can't remember exactly what that particular expression looks like! But they picked up on it and my aunty was nice about it, but kind of told me I needed to get that checked out as I didn't want to wait too long. I had only just turned twenty-six but she put the fear of God in me that time was a-tickin'.

It was not that long after this visit that I suddenly hit a wall and told my husband we had to move. I had tried to find a job close to home, but there was just nothing decent around. I had gone to a few interviews but nothing had come from them. In the end I just wasn't feeling the area that we lived in. I think a part of this feeling was that it was close to where I had lived as a teenager when my dad died, and it reminded me of that time in my life. My husband liked the area but I just never really felt connected there. To me it was actually a bit of a hole and I wanted to move to a bigger, more exciting new area.

Once I hit the wall and said I wasn't happy sitting on the train and couldn't do the long commute anymore, everything happened very quickly. We put our house on the market, bought a new house in an area we had liked for a while that was much closer to the city, my husband got a transfer at work to a new location twenty minutes from home and my train trip to the city was halved. We were in a beautiful suburb where there were lots of walking paths, gardens, lakes and shops. This place was so much nicer than the old hole.

However, after a few months, the excitement of being in a new house and area subsided and that longing to belong crept back in. But instead of joining a local sporting group, I changed jobs, and I changed jobs again, and again and again and again.

I had been in my very first job out of college for seven years, but after moving house, within the next twelve months I changed jobs five times. From not being able to find a job in my previous suburb to suddenly having lots of new jobs was a different feeling for me. I don't even think that I really wanted a new job in the first place, but I just liked the excitement of being offered a job. I think I was searching for that new place to belong in. And because the mothers group was closed as I didn't have a baby, I thought I would find a new tribe by finding the perfect new job. Yet really, I was looking externally to fill that void within.

## OWN YOUR TRUTH

I'm not usually the first person in a group to say the *Look at me, I'm awesome!* kind of thing. However, after being on the baby making train for a while, I kind of just let my "I've got everything sorted out" guard down—but just a little, and only to my closest family and friends. When I let my sisters and close friends in on my struggles, I felt very open and raw in the moment but also it felt magically freeing.

In this journey of belonging or not belonging, it is really when you tell your truth and show your vulnerability that you can start to let go. Even if just slightly. My vulnerability started to show only a little. However, it was a step in the right direction to belonging.

True belonging starts within ourselves. Instead of searching for external quick fixes that will make you feel good for a while, truly looking within yourself opens your heart, it frees the old, negative self-doubt and in doing so it makes room for new experiences.

When I was in my mid to late twenties, I never knew anyone who was going through infertility. There was no Facebook nor search engines to make life easier. I was given a pamphlet from the fertility centre and my details were put down on the mailing list.

So in the mail arrived this infertility newsletter with real-life stories and the latest medical information, and it had an upcoming events page. The fertility centre offered regular coffee and chat meet-ups for their patients all over the city.

These were hosted by one of the infertility clients. So I thought to myself, *I should really go to one of these one day.*

A few months passed and one Saturday off I drove to a suburb I had never been in before. I walked into a cafe and met a group of ladies on the baby making train, same as me.

It was bloody scary walking into that cafe, I was by myself and I didn't know anyone. I didn't even have a face to recognise. All I had was to try to find a table that had a teddy bear sitting on it, that was the identifying object. Otherwise it would have been like a blind date, awkwardly asking people if they were there to meet me.

However, once I got over the scary step of walking into that cafe and locating the teddy bear table, I sat and talked to women who were in similar situations as myself, trying to have a baby. It was so refreshing, all this time I had thought I was the only one going through this frustration and sadness. But I wasn't, and it was so refreshing, like a weight had been lifted from me. Each person had their own story or medical challenge, but we were joined by a similar yearning.

Afterwards, I drove home happy that I had taken that first step towards freeing myself of this silent struggle and I felt comforted that I wasn't the only person in the whole wide world suffering from infertility and going crazy.

After having the courage to put myself out there for that first meeting, I read in the next newsletter that there was a new coffee and chat coming up in my very own suburb. Wow, this must have been meant to be. And this particular event invited us to bring our partners, so it wasn't just for women like most of the events were.

So off I dragged my husband and we went to our local Coffee Club. And the whole "bring your partner along" thing didn't work, as not one of the other women had brought their husbands. However, my husband happily-ish stayed for half of it; he pretty much drank his coffee and when we girls started talking about cycles, he bailed. But I stayed on and at this one meet-up I met some amazing women. We were just a small group but we clicked, so I finally found my mothers group!

Well, my version of it anyway.

We all had different stories, but all experienced very similar emotions whilst on the baby making train.

From that point onwards we would organise to meet up, grab a coffee and have a catch-up chat on where we all were at on our journeys. This felt fantastic as I could just be myself. I didn't have to hide my struggles in silence. I could get advice on doctors and alternative therapies and hear the latest news. Letting go, being vulnerable and releasing the shame of failing to conceive a child was so freeing.

I would always come away from those chats with my close group more positive because I wasn't the only one in the whole world going through this.


## READ UP

Another thing that helped me was to read about women who were not following the normal pattern of child bearing and rearing. And when I started reading these stories, more would appear, making me think that having children isn't the pinnacle for all women and we are no less of a woman for not having them.

Jennifer Aniston said in her *HuffPost* article:

> Here's where I come out on this topic: we are complete with or without a mate, with or without a child. We get to decide for ourselves what is beautiful when it comes to our bodies. That decision is ours and ours alone. Let's make that decision for ourselves and for the young women in this world who look to us as examples. Let's make that decision consciously, outside of the tabloid noise. We don't need to be married or mothers to be complete. We get to determine our own "happily ever after" for ourselves.

There really are many amazing women in the public eye who have not had children for whatever reason and they don't seem to be suffering from a lack of belonging or purpose. Yes, some are very high-powered women, such as Oprah Winfrey, Ellen DeGeneres, Betty White, Helen Mirren and Kylie Minogue, and also many politicians. However, when you really look, there are many in your local area as well, though you may not have realised. In my corporate circle of friends there are some who every weekend raise money for animal shelters by sewing goods and selling them online, others volunteer at sporting events, sell raffles tickets for charities, run in events to raise money, and cook goodies on the weekends for fundraisers.

So, when you are struggling to find your "belonging" group, when you just want to be accepted into the mothers group but the doors are closed, you need to put yourself out there and open your own doors. If you want to you can open them completely wide, but even just a crack is a start. Open them to your closest family and friends, let them in on your personal struggles to conceive. Be authentic; it is so freeing, like a weight lifted right off your shoulders. Start your own group by getting out to a meet-up with women in similar shoes as you.

When you open this door a little, the wind will blow it right open and you will then feel the wind in your hair and openness in your heart.

# staying sane tips

1. *Open yourself up. Start with your closest family and friends. No one is perfect and when you open the door to vulnerability you might be surprised to receive more back.*

2. *True belonging is within ourselves. Instead of looking outwards for quick material fixes, turn within for self-reflection. You will learn so much more about yourself.*

3. *Put yourself out there by going to infertility group meet-ups. Yes, it can be daunting at first to walk into a room of strangers, but* everyone else is in the same boat initially. The experience *will greatly help you feel a sense of belonging.*

4. *Be your authentic self, it is so freeing.*

5. *Google and read about amazing women who do not have children for whatever reason. You might be surprised how many inspiring women there are and what they have done with their lives.*

# 3

# *That question*
# —getting the third degree

That question ... how many times have you been asked *that* question? You know the one well, it comes with many different facial expressions, sideways glances, held breaths, a quick search down your body for a hint of a slightly rounded belly. Sneaky questions asked to your mother, your sisters, your friends ... always trying to find out when they can expect to hear the pitter patter of tiny feet. We all want to hear the pitter patter but bloody hell, where are the tiny feet hiding?

How many times have you been asked that question? *So, when are you going to have kids? When are you going to start a family? Oh, upgrading your car to a four door ... are you getting ready for a baby? Oh, you have bought a new house, have you set aside one of the rooms for a nursery? You have been married now for a while ... when can we expect to start knitting baby booties?*

Or the remarks and comments like: *You both look so good holding little Johnny, it suits you! This room will make a great nursery. Oh, I'm getting rid of little Johnny's baby stuff, when shall I drop it over to your place? Because you'll be next! I thought you guys would have had kids by now. Everyone in the office seems to be pregnant, there must be something in the water here. I just had to look at my husband and I got pregnant. Oh, you two are going on a holiday, you might come home with a bun in the oven. You work too much, you should really slow down and plant some roots, like a family of your own. Kids just love you, you should hurry up and start a family.*

If that's not bad enough, there are the more-impersonal banks and insurance companies, even the census every five years. *Do you have any children? How many dependents do you have?* And the online forms, *Click this box if you have any children* and it opens up another box with *How many children do you have?*

The question is everywhere. I have been asked this question so many times that I have completely lost count. I was even asked this question at work by my previous manager in a performance review. 'Are you planning on having a family?' I was married and in my early thirties, so I think people saw that question as fair game. I answered a little awkwardly with a surprised and slightly pained look on my face: that is a complicated area. I think they read between the lines that all wasn't well in that department.

And what about the disappointment look? My husband and I went to a family friend's place to have lunch and there was a gathering of people who he had spent his teenage years around. And as soon as we walked in, I got the look … that look of disappointment. They even looked behind me, trying to see a small child following us into the house. And I could just hear them thinking … *Why haven't they had children?*

Then out it came: 'You guys haven't had kids yet?' in a disapproving tone of voice. It wasn't really even a question, more like an expression of disapproval at us *choosing* to not have kids.

The lunch followed and I felt like I was not involved in the conversation as it was all about kids. It felt like I was a leper or had some kind of disease, when really I am a human with purpose, regardless of how many dependents I may or may not have.

I did actually make it to dessert, but straight after that I was like *Get me out of here. Never to return!*

I was at a lovely post-meeting lunch with the business partners. I was at a table with only women and out of the six of us I was the only one without children, and as per many times before, I got the *So do you have any kids?* question (what now seems like on cue). And I'm such an old hand at this question now I said, 'No, I don't have any kids,' and I can see their facial expressions, their searching faces trying to work out why I wouldn't have kids as they do. And when I see their searching faces that are trying to work out something in common with me, I then said 'But I have my niece living with us at the moment, she is studying and trying to save up money to go overseas.' And I share a funny story about that experience to show that I have something in common.

Other times when I answer with the *No, I don't have kids* line and again see the curiosity on their faces followed by a long pause, I throw in that I have a dog and tell a funny story about animals. Or explain that I have lots of nieces and nephews.

Also, there always seems to be the *You'll be next* comment. Why is it that many well-intending family and friends assume that once a couple is married or have been together for a set number of years that they automatically will have children? And that they have the right to ask this question or comment.

And baby showers can be the worst.

I have been to all the baby showers. How many times have you smelt the chocolate-filled nappies, guessed the date/time/weight/sex of the baby and played pass the parcel with the nursery themed wrapping paper around the circle of women, all while happily smiling and chatting? Some I've been to were enjoyable, as I was able to catch up with friends and enjoy a glass of champagne, but others were OTT, where there were many young mums with bumps or babies everywhere.

At the baby showers you're been to—with the rooms full of women and all the baby talk—how many times have you deflected *that* question?

How do you answer the question without hyperventilating or babbling on about the weather—without sculling the wine and avoiding Aunty Mary, who now thinks you have an alcohol problem?

Answer: the truth!

The truth shall set you free, right? You have probably heard that so many times before. But do you feel that you can really tell the truth in this situation? This one is a biggie and will take time. So please give that to yourself.

Just start off by only telling the truth in situations where you feel completely comfortable. Close family and friends is where you start to tell the truth. They might just surprise you and help you immensely. And it can really help with not having to scull that bottle of wine before going to the barbecue. Also, if possible, tell your story in one-on-one conversations as it won't be so daunting.

Being truthful with your "hoping to have a baby but it's taking its sweet ass time" with your close family and friends will feel like a weight has been lifted off your shoulders. You might actually enjoy going to the family barbecue and they may provide some great relief from the burden of being on the baby-making train ride. A problem shared is a problem solved—this might not completely work in this particular situation, but the "problem solved" part might just be that you don't feel so alone anymore.

For me, it was a slow process of letting people in. Firstly with my sisters and a few of my closest friends. Opening up about my baby making struggles really helped me with that feeling of loneliness, as I had always seemed to think that I was the only one in the world struggling in this area. However, when I opened up to my closest I realised that I wasn't the only one and that others had struggles as well. When I would hear or read something new on getting pregnant, I would share this with them, and vice versa.

One of my closest was really struggling when she would walk down the street and just see pregnant bumps or babies everywhere. And I said to her, 'Instead of feeling frustrated at them, try to think to yourself that you will be next, that you will be the one walking down the street with the pregnant belly.' I tried to visualise this myself. And guess what? She *was* next and I also felt good because I think I helped on some level.

However, telling the truth will only work in situations where you feel comfortable. Getting asked *that* question when you are at the business partners' lunch meeting is probably not ideal as this is a professional setting. And yes, we talk about family in these situations, however usually just high-level information, not all the dramatic details. If you do not feel comfortable, the best answer is deflection or changing the subject.

Deflection could be as easy as answering with *Someday we will* or *Right now we are happy with just us two, but hopefully in the future*. It's all about common ground. These easy answers hint that you do actually want children, which is the truth for you and the common ground for the person asking the question. The light deflection of "someday" or "in the future" is still the truth but without all the nitty-gritty, or feelings of discomfort.

If the deflection is followed by *Well, don't leave it too long as the clock is ticking!* when you are not in your close family or close friends group, change the subject around by asking them questions about their kids. Asking questions is an easy option to take the spotlight off yourself.

And there is always humour. If you don't feel comfortable answering with the truth or with deflection, using humour is a light and fun way to answer. With humour you don't have to answer with a clear yes or no to whether you will have children. Answering with humour will simply turn the topic back to the person asking the question and as they will be laughing and answering a funny question from you, their train of thought will change direction.

How you answer will also depend on the situation—when and where you get asked the question. If you are sitting down to a Sunday lunch with the aunties and uncles and you get asked this question and everyone is staring at you, it's probably best to answer with humour and deflection. Really it is all about what you feel comfortable with telling.

Answering with the truth will come more easily with time and confidence within yourself, so don't be too hard on yourself at first.

I remember being at a family function when I was thirty and my aunty asked me if I was going to have kids, and I said yes, we hope to have kids one day. And she took that and said that it's great we are going travelling first (we had been on some overseas holidays) and she started talking about the fact that it can be harder to travel overseas once you have kids. And I just accepted her take on things and the conversation quickly changed to something else. However, when I was thirty-six, another aunty asked me the kid question and I said, 'I'm honestly not sure, we have tried and I have some medical issues.' This was the truth and she was completely lovely and offered support without pushing the "clock is ticking" point. It felt so nice and freeing being completely truthful.

Also, when you tell the truth you might be surprised to hear that many other people have had difficulty trying to conceive. And you would probably have never known this about them, and it could actually bring you closer together. It will increase your circle of friends to whom you can turn when you are on the infertility train ride.

Be kind to yourself and don't overthink it. We spend so much time worrying about what other people think of us, but at the end of the day they don't really think about us as much as we think they do!

# staying sane tips

1.  *When you stop hiding and deflecting family-barbecue baby conversations by telling the truth, it will feel like a weight has been lifted off your shoulders.*

2.  *Assess the situation. If you are asked* that *question at a business lunch meeting, best to deflect or change the subject. Or simply ask questions back, such as* What tips do you have for balancing work with raising small children? *This will deflect the question and you might get some key insights for when Baby comes along.*

3.  *Try easy deflection by answering* that *question with* Someday we will *or* Hopefully in the future. *This will give you common ground. You are answering truthfully and it will give you common ground for further discussion.*

4.  *If your easy-deflection answer is met with another, more probing question, such as the "ticking body clock" one, answer with humour, have a laugh and change the subject.*

5.  *Don't be too hard on yourself if you struggle with answering with the truth, as this will take time and confidence. However, the truth is very freeing.*

6.  *By answering with the truth, you might be surprised to hear that others have struggled to conceive, and you might get some handy tips on how they dealt with it.*

7.  *Don't worry about what other people think of you, as that is none of your business. And they really don't think about you as much as you might think they do.*

---

# 4

# Not all doctors are the same

Why do we treat doctors as godlike creatures? When we go to a fertility doctor, we see the word "specialist" and we treat them differently because their job title has the word "special" in it, right?

We sit directly opposite them, look at their gold-font medical plaques on the wall and think … they really are special. They walk into the room and as we hold our breath we feel like we could bow to them or curtsy. And we watch them like hawks, every word, every look, every eyebrow raise they have while reading our personal medical charts and results. We know that whatever they say is actually gold.

These fertility doctors have studied, trained and worked for many years to get that word "specialist" in their job title. Many early mornings, long nights and on-call weekends assisting patients. The hours and dedication are intense. And when you bring in the extremely emotional situation of new patients' desperation, these doctors really hold the key to our future.

But do they all hold the key to our future? And do they for every single case?

## THE GP

After we had moved house closer to the city so that I didn't have to commute on the horrible train for endless hours every day, we settled into our new life. After the craziness of house buying, selling and moving, changing jobs a few times, and finally getting a new job I was happy with etc., we went to our GP with our concerns about not falling pregnant. Our GP wanted us to get some basic tests done and for me that was the dreaded blood test.

Have I mentioned that I don't like doctors, pass out at the thought of blood tests, and am totally freaked out about hospitals? It's childhood trauma I'm sure from getting my tonsils out when I was five. The nurses had come at me during the night to jab me with a needle in my bum, resulting in my ongoing fear of needles. I remember suddenly getting woken up from a peaceful sleep with a heap of nurses surrounding my bed but my mother not there and having this needle come straight for me. I haven't had a tetanus shot or any other arm needles since I was thirteen years old and I'm now forty. So I will pretty much try to avoid needles and doctors and hospitals as that environment makes me anxious.

The first tests that a GP routinely requests require a blood test, so there just wasn't any way I could avoid this. I knew this day would come and I remember it so clearly. I walked into the test room and saw all the little red bottles of the recent samples the nurse had just taken. There was a light blue, padded chair with big, wide arms for you to rest your arm on. There was also a bed, but the nurse had all her paperwork over it. I was trying to be strong and just sat up on the big blue chair. The nurse looked at my arms and asked me to start pumping my hands to try and make my veins pop. She hmm'd and hrr'd a little as apparently I have small veins ... oh yay! Finally the needle went in and she quickly drew blood.

Before I knew it, the blood test had finished and I felt massive relief. I expected that one blood test would be the only blood test I would have to go through in my whole entire life. I got up from the big blue chair and walked out of that clinic smiling with my husband. However, as soon as I got to the street to walk across to the car, I nearly fainted. Suddenly I felt the blood drain out of me and I just could not stand up, let alone walk. There was a park bench nearby and I sat and completely slumped in it by lying down in my husband's lap. I must have looked like I had been partying the previous night, but after ten minutes I felt better and we drove home.

## THE OLD-FART DOCTOR

Our GP advised that our test results were all normal, my blood test and my husband's sperm test appeared fine. So we were referred to a fertility specialist in the city.

Off we trotted into the city with our hopefulness coming along for the ride. And what a ride it has turned out to be.

During our first IVF specialist encounter, I remember walking into the medical suites and the decor being very brown and drab. We sat down and patiently waited and when our names are called, we walked into the doctor's office and sat eagerly as he looked over our results and started his spiel.

This doctor had very grey hair and looked old and in my head I referred to him as the old-fart doctor. He didn't give any emotional comfort to us ... it was all business. All I remember from that meeting was him telling us that the ideal time to fall pregnant was between twenty-seven and thirty-four. And at the time I thought, *Awesome, I can run fast out the door of this old-fart doctor's office and just chill,* because I was only twenty-seven. I wanted to escape as the old-fart doctor was just reciting all the procedural details on fertility options in his very bland, businesslike manner.

As the old-fart doctor had scared me off with all his talk of blood tests and needles, we didn't do anything for the next ten months. So finally, after I had worked up the courage to call his office and take that next step, the receptionist advised that Old Fart was on extended holidays and I was referred to another doctor.

So when I was twenty-eight we went to see this new doctor, and he was just lovely. So kind and he was not scary at all.

## THE LOVELY DOCTOR

The lovely doctor recommended that I go on Clomid tablets first, which is an oral medication that stimulates ovulation, therefore guaranteeing that each month I would ovulate. He also suggested I have a procedure called a hysterosalpingogram, which is a special type of X-ray examination that checks for any blockages of the fallopian tubes and uterus. The entire test takes about forty-five minutes. During the procedure, a thin catheter is inserted through the cervix into the uterus, a special dye is injected and X-rays are taken of the dye.

So early one morning we drove off to the biggest hospital in the city. Even the car park was huge and we pulled into the very last parking space. We walked into one of the many entries and wandered around in circles for a while, and thankfully a volunteer saw us looking lost and walked us all the way to where we were supposed to go.

Again, I'm not a fan of hospitals. I was asked to fully undress and put on this lovely hospital gown. Next I was in the operating room with all these scary-looking medical instruments. I was told to sit up on a table and put my feet into stirrups, and that this procedure is done while I'm fully awake, no anaesthetic for this. The nurses had absolutely no friendly or comforting words at all, I just had to obey their instructions.

So I was in this operating room with all the sterile objects and bright fluorescent lights, with my feet in stirrups and no clothes on, just lying there for all the world to see whilst being completely awake. They injected the coloured dye up into my fallopian tubes, and took photos to see if there were any blockages.

I hadn't had any hospital procedures since I was a child, when my tonsils were removed, and this was a horrible experience. The strange doctors and nurses had no warmth, not even distracting small talk. I felt like an object, like I was their last patient at the end of a long shift. I walked as fast as

I could out of that hospital thinking … is a baby really worth this?

The results from this lovely procedure came back all fine.

Before I knew it, I had turned thirty years old and as the Clomid tablets hadn't magically made me pregnant, the next step was to do the IUI procedure. IUI stands for intrauterine insemination, which is when they take the sperm and wash and spin it, then place it inside the woman's uterus at ovulation. This hopefully increases the number of sperm that reach the fallopian tubes, subsequently increasing the chance of fertilisation.

Normally, to find out if a woman is ovulating, the fertility clinic recommends that a blood test be done each morning around the middle of the month for a few consecutive days. However, I expressed my issues with blood tests and Lovely Doctor said that I could instead do ovulation tests at home, which means peeing on a stick first thing in the morning. OMG, what a relief, as the thought of driving into the city very early each morning and getting a blood test sparked panic within me. I could feel the inclination to run for the hills and escape this nightmare.

So I jumped onto eBay and bought a super pack of one hundred ovulation tests from China. I was ready, set and just waiting for the pee stick test to give me the go signal.

Ok so what does one do when the ovulation test shows a positive "go" day and it's a weekend? Yep, our first IUI and the ovulation day was a Sunday. *Great,* I thought, *that means I have to inconvenience the lovely doctor on a Sunday.*

However, I got a bit mixed up on the instructions.

I had my positive ovulation test, the hubby had his sperm in a plastic container wrapped in a brown paper bag and off we went on our Sunday drive into the city. We dropped off the sperm sample and I lined up for a blood test to confirm that I was definitely ovulating. The lab then washed and spun the sperm and my blood test results came back confirming I was ovulating.

We took the lift up to the lovely doctor floor, but the clinic was closed. So we called Lovely Doctor on the weekend telephone number and said we were ready and waiting at his clinic. He said that we should have called him early this morning as he now had to drop what he was doing and quickly drive into the clinic, as there was only a short window of time left before sperm was no longer good.

Oops, I had assumed that the blood test or lab nurses would call the doctor to come in if it's a weekend, but we were supposed to. On reading the weekend instructions more closely, it definitely said: *If it's your body clock, you ring the doc.*

Why couldn't I have ovulated one day later, on a Monday? That is convenient for everyone, right? I felt really bad for our lovely doctor, what if it were his wife's or kid's birthday and I was the one tearing him away from his weekend family time? All for an eight per cent increased chance of me falling pregnant?

However, our lovely doctor still lived up to his nickname, he was still lovely to us on that Sunday.

We went on to do four IUIs with Lovely Doctor, all of which were unsuccessful. I'd get my hopes up, and think to myself

... *Maybe I'm pregnant!* However, it always seemed to come crashing down.

The next step on from IUIs is of course the big one ... in vitro fertilisation, or IVF. The one where you hear all the stories of how invasive and expensive it is and the drugs make you go crazy, and that it's an emotional roller-coaster. We had heard the stories but decided to sign up for it anyway, simply in the hope of getting the chance to hold our own baby.

We just thought that, with IVF, it absolutely works, how could it not? They would take lots of my eggs out, and select under a microscope my husband's best sperm and inject it into my eggs. Then they would grow the fertilised eggs for five days and put the best-looking ones back in, right up into my uterus. And the embryo then would do its thing by implanting into my uterus wall, where it would grow for nine months and then I would give birth to our baby.

So this had to work, all my body had to do was grow lots of good eggs and implant the fertilised embryo into my uterus wall.

Just before we were about to start our very first IVF cycle, my husband and I were snuggling on the couch one night and he said to me that he was super excited. We were finally doing something that would bring our baby to us. Because we absolutely thought IVF worked.

## THE KIND DOCTOR

Naturally, as we really liked our lovely doctor, we were just about to start IVF with him. However, the naturopath we had been seeing for the last two years—a well-known Chinese medicine fertility expert very experienced in the IVF world—strongly advised us to go to this new and more modern clinic instead.

With IVF, you have your doctors clinic, and they use a separate pathology team and separate hospital for the egg retrieval procedure. Therefore, you have to go to about three different medical suites for your consultations and procedures.

I had never given any thought to IVF clinics, I had just assumed that there was one big clinic in each city that everyone went to. Little did I know there were actually lots of different clinics. And because we completely trusted our naturopath, we changed clinics from the lovely doctor to the new modern clinic.

Firstly, we went to an open night at the clinic where they gave us all the information and we had a look around the rooms and even did a tour of their onsite embryo laboratory. At the info night they also provided cheese and crackers, so it was a fun night out on the town for us, really … not!

With my fear of hospitals, this new clinic was amazing. The previous clinic had used a big hospital in a completely different building for the egg retrieval procedure, which I didn't like the sound of. Instead, the new clinic had modern decor, comfy couches, TV, and a food-and-drink counter. So, if I had to come in for a scan in the middle of the day during the working week, I could grab lunch there as well, like my very own mini buffet. And the hospital for the egg retrieval was five steps outside the clinic reception area, therefore it had its own private hospital suite. This was comforting to me as it had that homely feel to it.

At the new clinic, my doctor was really kind. In her office she had photos on her desk of her four gorgeous children. This made me feel hopeful.

Over the next eight months, at thirty-one years old, I did four embryo transfers, but only three with Kind Doctor. For my very first embryo transfer, which is usually about five days after you have the egg retrieval procedure, the transfer day fell on a weekend. *What! Again? I'm inconveniencing a doctor on a weekend!* And this particular weekend was a long weekend. My kind doctor had the weekend off, so the founding doctor of the clinic did my transfer that Saturday morning.

## THE NO-FILTER DOCTOR

We had never met this doctor before and he was completely different from Kind Doctor … he was more of a "say the first thing that comes into your mind" doctor. Let's call him No-Filter Doctor.

So No-Filter Doctor walked into the embryo transfer room, looked at my husband and asked him if he was a police officer, commenting on his height because he is tall. He didn't really say much to me, no nice encouraging words even though it was my very first embryo transfer, which was a huge deal for me. However, what he did talk about was his holiday home up the coast, where he was going to drive afterwards and spend the weekend. He was whinging about the gardener there, complaining that they may not have cleaned up the gardens properly before their arrival.

So I was lying there with an ultrasound device scanning my stomach, legs wide for the world to see, and No-Filter Doctor, whom I had never met before, was whinging about his holiday home. And I thought to myself, is this really happening? It was like an out-of-body experience and I felt a bit like an object that had to get processed before knock-off time.

After doing these four rounds of IVF—with the last one being unsuccessful again, as I found out on Christmas morning when I woke up with my period—we decided to have a break. It was taking over our life, all the scheduling and appointments, and we just wanted to get back to fun and adventure.

So in the January after that unsuccessful IVF Christmas, when I turned thirty-two years old, we took that year off. And over that Christmas and New Year holiday season, my friend and I came up with a motto for the year: it was going to be The Year of "Anything Goes".

You know when New Year's comes around and you excitedly think of all the possibilities the year will bring? For me, I was always just wanting a baby. But if I wasn't going to do IVF, I wasn't going to get my baby, therefore, what else could I want?

As the previous Christmas had sucked, I wanted our next Christmas to be amazing. So my "anything goes" friend and I suggested that we have a white Christmas. (We had enjoyed a few drinks at the time of coming up with this crazy idea, and I thought everything was a great idea!)

But after the holiday season, January slips into February and before you know it it's early March already. Because I wasn't doing any IVF, I didn't have any life plans or goals, it was just a mundane "going to work five days a week" kind of thing.

In early March, one weeknight I had gone to bed but kept thinking about my motto of "anything goes" and having an awesome white Christmas to block out the memory of the last Christmas. So I got out of bed and went to my computer and sent my friend a message; as they lived in Far North Queensland and had a three-year-old child, I didn't want to ring them and wake up the house. The message said 'Let's do that white Christmas this year!' And I went back to bed and dreamed about a white Christmas. The next morning I excitedly checked my messages, no reply. And there was no reply all day, but finally the next night I received a reply that said 'Ok, let's do this.' Our husbands were on board and the next eight months were spent planning our white Christmas holiday to Canada and the USA. This gave me purpose and a feeling of such excitement. I could plan something and *actually get it*, unlike with IVF—I could plan that but I never actually got it.

We had planned that once we got home from our big white Christmas adventure I would do some more IVF embryo transfers, as I had two in the freezer. However, even the best of plans can go out the door.

On the third day of our three-week white Christmas adventure, my husband decided that he could ski like he was at the Winter Olympics and his first run down the mountain ended with him being ambulanced to the nearest hospital. Maybe he should have had that refresher course! He fractured his knee and was on crutches for the rest of our holiday.

Once we got home, there was no way he could return to his new job—which he had only just got four months before we went to Canada—as it was in the mines doing very physical work. So our plans for another embryo transfer were put back in the freezer.

My husband had to rethink what he wanted to do with his career. His knee was not recovering and he definitely could not do physical work, so he went back to university to study for a new career less demanding on the body. And the knee injury recovery took another two years. So there went my plans of motherhood at thirty-three and also thirty-four.

## THE THERAPIST

After we had these few years on break from IVF and mending broken bones, I was feeling the need to get back onto the baby making train. But I felt that I needed to mend myself mentally beforehand.

At IVF clinics they briefly mention counselling, it is like an afterthought and most people, including myself at first, just shrug off that suggestion and act all tough. However, I felt like I needed to speak with a professional, but more as a precaution or to be proactive rather than reactive. There was a counsellor advertised in our local rag who every week wrote a column helping people who wrote in with their issues. So I made a booking to go and speak with her. It was actually quite good, we spoke about IVF and parenting. She used to be a midwife so was really experienced in this area. However, at the end of our first session she suggested I may need to go on antidepressants. This was a bit of a shock to me as I had never considered this, nor had any of my doctors. I felt really good, and was seeing her more as a precaution for my next IVF cycle.

So two weeks later I went back to see her and we were talking and at the end of our session she advised that I didn't need antidepressants, which was great, as I hadn't wanted them to start with! It was a bit of an eye opener for me as she was so willing to hand them out. However, I am more of a person who prefers to heal myself naturally from within. And also with IVF I was already putting so much medication into my body, that I didn't want any more.

## THE INVESTIGATIVE DOCTOR

When my husband was home recovering from his second knee operation, which took place a few months short of two years post Canada, he had to have six weeks on crutches with no driving. During this time I saw a new IVF clinic open in my very own suburb, which I thought was a sign! I wouldn't have to battle peak-hour traffic to drive into the big city. And as the hubby was home recovering, I thought now was a great time to go visit a new clinic.

So with not having done any fertility stuff in years, off we went to see this new doctor in our home suburb. I walked into the doctor's room followed by my husband who walked in on crutches. Our new doctor made a funny comment: 'You know

I'm a fertility doctor, not a knee doctor?'

I had gone into super-organised mode and brought copies of all my old records, tests, egg retrieval numbers, embryo photos, etc. The doctor was reading through my paperwork and straight away saw something that no other doctor had ever picked up on before—that the very first test I had had that checked the tubes and uterus showed something. Wow, that test had been done when I was thirty, before I had done any IVF cycles. And now I was nearly thirty-five years old.

I liked this new doctor straight away … when you know, you know! So he became Investigative Doctor. He saw stuff that others before him hadn't seen.

So just after I turned thirty-five, he booked me in for a laparoscopy and hysteroscopy.

A laparoscopy is a very common keyhole surgery performed for fertility patients via a small cut in the abdomen where they can view the interior of the abdominal or pelvic cavities and see what's going on inside. They check the reproductive organs and pelvis for abnormal deposits of endometrial tissue, scarring or cysts and, if appropriate, remove this tissue from the organs.

A hysteroscopy is a procedure that allows the doctor to examine the cervix and look inside the uterus using a thin, lighted telescope that is inserted into the vagina. This is where my new doctor had seen something on my old scan. He removed a large polyp from my uterus; this polyp may have hindered my previous embryo transfers from implanting into the uterus wall.

He discovered that I had adenomyosis and a very little bit of endometriosis.

Adenomyosis occurs when the cells that normally line the uterus also grow in the layer of muscle in the wall of the uterus, therefore potentially stopping an embryo from implanting. Endometriosis occurs when the tissue lining of the uterus, called the endometrium, grows outside of the uterus.

The only way to completely remove adenomyosis is to have a hysterectomy, but as I was only thirty-five years old and hadn't had kids, I didn't exactly fancy that. So our doctor recommended we shrink the adenomyosis with a medication treatment called Zoladex.

Over the next five months I had a monthly Zoladex implant injected just under the skin near the belly button to try to reduce the adenomyosis. Again, this was a needle in my stomach, but I was getting used to needles and medical procedures.

After the five implants—which sent my body into a mini menopausal state (hello hot flushes during winter!)—I did an embryo transfer. I had two frozen embryos from my previous clinic and who knew that you can actually move embryos from one clinic to the next? You just have to sign the paperwork and order the courier driver … that easy.

The frozen embryo transfer was unsuccessful, which was really disappointing as I had gone through the investigative surgery and the five months of implant injections and hot flushes. However, my investigative doctor wanted to run a different blood test and this test came back showing that I had a blood disorder. Again, more investigative doctor stuff … he should really be a medical detective.

This blood disorder is hereditary, and the test even

pinpointed that it is only from one parent, not both. And as my father had already passed away, I assumed it was from his side. In general day-to-day life this blood disorder is not a big deal, but the blood specialist that we went to see on a two-hour drive away said that I simply have a higher chance of blood clots. The blood disorder also means that I have a higher chance of second-trimester miscarriage. Therefore, if I were to fall pregnant I would need to take an injection daily from week thirteen to six weeks after I give birth. Yay for me, who doesn't like needles. But I would have done it if meant I could finally hold my baby.

So my last frozen embryo transfer was in November and I saw the blood disorder doctor in January, around my thirty-sixth birthday, and I went to call my awesome investigative doctor in February to get the ball rolling again as I still had one frozen embryo waiting. On speaking with the receptionist, she mentioned that my awesome investigative doctor was retiring. What the! We had a thing going on and it was amazing, and another woman told me that he was leaving me! The receptionist said he was only taking final appointments, so I quickly booked myself in to see him as I was heartbroken and needed closure.

So I again left work early one day to see my awesome investigative doctor for one last time by myself and he told me it wasn't me, but him. That the time had come for him to spend time with his family. He gave me a referral for another doctor who was part of the same clinic, but there was nothing in my suburb anymore. I'd have to drive one hour to see this new doctor.

During my last rendezvous with my awesome investigative doctor, I asked him everything I could possibly think of. A close family friend had mentioned to me that she would be a surrogate and carry my child. Wow, that is such a big thing and I am still so grateful to her. So I asked my awesome investigative doctor about this as our relationship was ready for it and he gave me the lowdown on all things surrogacy in Australia, which is very limited. *Oh, but I have read in the celebrity magazines that Nicole Kidman and Sarah Jessica Parker have done it!* I thought. *Oh, but wait, they are in the USA and have mega bucks to afford it.*

Surrogacy in Australia is extremely hard. You would think that with such a small population compared to other countries that we would make it easier for the everyday person, but this is not so.

In Australia you cannot pay someone to have your baby, only cover their medical bills. And as they are giving birth to the child, on the birth certificate they are the legal mother, even though it may not be their own embryo. Therefore, the biological mother needs to adopt their own child.

Oh, and my awesome investigative doctor gave me the paperwork and at the time in early 2014 it was twenty thousand dollars for one embryo transfer, as there is no Medicare coverage. He also advised that a number of IVF clinics will not perform surrogacy procedures if that clinic is linked to a religious hospital, as certain religions do not believe in surrogacy. There goes my Catholic upbringing.

## THE HAPPY TRANSFER DOCTOR

So off we went to another IVF specialist, this time in another hospital clinic that we had to locate and find parking at and whose general layout we had to familiarise ourselves with.

We met our new doctor, who I called Happy Transfer Doctor. He read over our paperwork and as I had become my own specialist at seeing lots of different doctors, I asked the questions. He was a happy, funny doctor and we really liked his easygoing nature.

So only one month after I had broken up with my previous doctor, my new happy transfer doctor wanted me to get back on the bandwagon straight away. At this meeting he asked me what day of my cycle I was on and as I was at the beginning, he booked me in for an embryo transfer the following weekend, as I still had one last embryo waiting in the freezer.

So our relationship with Happy Transfer Doctor kicked off quickly and with a bang. We saw him the following week for our last embryo transfer, which again was unsuccessful.

It was a weird feeling not having any embryos left in the freezer, as I was now thirty-six and had had embryos stored since I was thirty-one. It's like a safety blanket, a comfy feeling, knowing that they are there for a rainy day.

We took the next few months off and partied, went camping and went out in the city. Just enjoyed being normal.

That May I started googling natural fertility programs again and we signed up for a full-body detox through this naturopath. So from June to November we both lost weight, were exercising daily and eating super healthy; we were on the best supplements and taking homeopathic treatments.

In November I went in for a fresh IVF cycle. I hadn't done a fresh cycle in five years. And because we were super healthy, we produced the best and most amazing embryos ever ... and I was five years older. Also, it helped that I wasn't stressed by the process as I knew what to expect.

I had a fresh embryo transferred, but yet again it was unsuccessful. And as this was early December now, we just relaxed over Christmas and partied through New Year's. In February we went to see Happy Transfer Doctor as I had just turned thirty-seven and was feeling like I should keep going. I discussed my body concerns with him, that after I have an embryo transfer I never ever make it through the two-week wait, I always have a full-on period before the two weeks are up—which you are not supposed to. But he just wanted me to go in for another transfer, as I was lucky to now have five in the freezer. But it just didn't feel right to me; though I had expressed my concerns, his answer was just more transfers, therefore more money for him.

This kind of put me off for a while and for that whole year I never went back to see Happy Transfer Doctor. During that year we just partied, did fun stuff and had work commitments and doing an embryo transfer just wasn't high on my list. I think I was getting discouraged and my feelings of wanting to have a baby were weakening. I was just enjoying myself with lots of other non-baby stuff ... such as living in the now.

The whole year of me being thirty-seven and not doing any

transfers nearly turned into a whole year of me being thirty-eight and not doing any transfers. In the second half of my thirty-eighth year I had thoughts of doing a transfer, just to give it a shot, as I had to keep paying for the frozen embryo storage every six months.

However, shit happened in that my husband had a work accident, where he fell and broke his collarbone and fractured his neck. So he was in a sling and neck brace for three months with no work and no driving. And the embryo thoughts went completely out the door. He took his neck brace off three days before Christmas and the next January, when I turned thirty-nine, thoughts of embryos were still out the door.

## THE EXPERT DOCTOR

In June of that year, with my husband back at work and mostly recovered, I went online and started researching IVF doctors, which I had never done before. The IVF doctors we had gone to were all advised to us by our GP or naturopath or referred by other IVF specialists. We had never done our own research, let alone asked for a specific doctor.

I found that there was another clinic and a particular doctor who specialised in my exact issue: adenomyosis. His speciality in this field was serious, as he was on medical boards and had written papers, etc. This was amazing: finally, a doctor who knew about my adenomyosis.

I called the clinic, which was in the city (as they usually are) and the receptionist advised that this doctor did fortnightly consults at the medical suites in my very own suburb. *OMG, it's a sign!* So I booked us in to see him one Friday afternoon a few weeks later.

My husband and I both drove straight from work and met at the local clinic. My expectations on arrival were that we would rock up at reception, sit down for an hour and wait, because that is what you do at medical suites. However, when we walked up to the counter and were asked to fill in the standard form, waiting behind the counter was our new doctor. He was smiling and having a joke with us to write quicker. There was no sitting down and waiting for ages. This doctor greeted us on entry with a smile and a joke … it was like gold-class service.

Once we were seated in the doctor's office, he went through our records and asked lots of questions. I also asked him lots of questions and told him my concerns. This expert doctor knew everything about my adenomyosis condition, he knew way more than I did. So much so that on a blank piece of paper he wrote out seven action steps that he would advise for us. Things we had never been advised of before. He also took notes for the receptionist to photocopy information journals for us to read.

It was comforting that he knew so much about my condition. And when I mentioned that we had been to a few doctors during our time and had been moved around because doctors were retiring etc., he joked that he would not be retiring for a while.

We left our new expert doctor with a spring in our step, thinking of all possibilities. Expert Doctor gave us so much information we needed to start reading up on.

What a difference time and experience can make. When I first started seeing an IVF doctor, I was only twenty-seven years old and so young and wide eyed and just sat there listening to every word they said. So different to when I was thirty-nine and doing my own research online, reviewing my records and asking a heap of questions.

With the different types of IVF doctors … you name them, we have seen them. From the original Old-Fart Doctor, to Lovely Doctor, Kind Doctor, No-Filter Doctor, Investigative Doctor, Happy Transfer Doctor to Expert Doctor. We have been to their clinics, got friendly with the receptionist team, even found out where the best parking spots and coffee places are.

For anyone who does not like blood tests or has small veins, the best things you can do are to drink a heap of water before you go, this helps make your veins pop, and stay warm; if it is winter take a heat pack with you and sit it on both of your arms. Ask to lay down in the blood room, none of this sitting in the big blue chair and fainting afterwards. Even if they have their paperwork all over the bed. I now lie down every single time and can easily walk out and drive afterwards. And when they are about to draw the blood, talk heaps to the nurse taking the blood or think of something else very quickly. I used to think I was at a concert, standing on the floor, and I would feel the music and beat. This always worked as I love music and concerts.

More on needles: if you don't like injecting yourself for the hormone injections try to have your partner or a close friend who is good with needles learn how to inject them for you. An easy spot is the stomach area. Try relaxing on the couch and watch some silly TV show to try to tune your mind out to the fact that a big needle may just go into your belly. Rest your stomach and focus on the TV—it will be over before you know it.

Doctors are not gods, they are only human, just like us. Ask all the questions; if you think of it, ask them. If you think of questions when you get home, email them. It is better to get clarity than have it playing over and over in your mind.

Question their treatment plans. When you are starting out you will pretty much follow exactly what they advise as you don't yet know how your body will react to the medication. But after your first round you will know. And with medications there are usually other brands that do the same thing, but different bodies can react to a certain brand of medication better. Know this stuff, write it down or get photocopies from the receptionist or nurses.

Also keep a track of your own IVF cycles, just a quick and easy Google Sheet of what you took, how much and on what days of your cycle and which months of the year. This will be very handy if you have to do a few cycles—or if you are successful early on with a bouncing baby, and want to give them a sibling—as it is so easy to forget all the medications, dosages, days of the cycle, etc.

No one else knows your body and cycle as you do. So, if you are going through an IVF cycle, keep a journal for yourself of your symptoms, reactions and emotions. There will be so much going through your head that it is much better to get it down in a small journal. This will go well with keeping track of your cycle, days and medications.

When it comes to choosing an IVF clinic and doctor, it may feel like there are so many to choose from. Ask your GP for at least two or three that they recommend. And if you have the time, go and see at least two IVF doctors at different clinics. This will help you make a decision on which doctor and clinic is the best fit for you. When you are fresh to the world of IVF you may think that all clinics and doctors are the same, but they are very different. Some are at big hospitals whereas others are standard clinics.

Also, if you know you have a particular fertility issue, ask your GP for a specialist in that area. Or do it yourself, go online and research doctors that specialise in your concern. By doing this you are in control, and you will also find that there are specialists out there just for you.

Otherwise, ask your IVF friends or naturopath contacts if they can recommend any names. However, be aware of doctor review websites. These can give you a headache, as anyone can put anything online. When I found my expert doctor, the reviews of him online were fifty-fifty. And to the extreme, with one review absolutely loving him, and the next review not favourable at all. I had never reviewed a doctor online before and when I went to my first appointment, I was not sure which way it was going to go. I was pleasantly surprised.

Get a doctor who is doing it for the passion, not the money. Money ones will just want to keep doing transfer after transfer without investigating. Because I was thirty-one at first, I think the doctors thought I would be easy and didn't really look into my tube test, however when I was thirty-five and saw that different doctor, time was getting away from me and he looked more into my "why". Find a doctor that you both feel comfortable with, as it will be a crazy ride.

# staying sane tips

1. *For blood tests, drink plenty of water beforehand and stay calm, lie down and in your mind take yourself to your happy place.*

2. *For hormone injections, keep your stomach muscles very relaxed and distract yourself by watching something silly on TV. The needle will be over before you know it.*

3. *When seeing your doctor, ask lots of questions. If you forget to ask something, email them.*

4. *You know your body the best, so let your doctor know exactly what is normal with your body and if you are not reacting as per the medication, tell them and ask for a different brand of medication.*

5. *Keep a calendar of your cycle dates, medications and dosages and write in a journal how you are feeling, your symptoms and emotions.*

6. *Ask your GP for a number of fertility specialists and clinic recommendations.*

7. *Visit at least two fertility clinics to get a look and feel for your best match.*

8.  *If you have a specific fertility issue, search for a doctor who specialises in this area, as their treatment plan will be better suited.*

9.  *Find a doctor who you connect with and feel comfortable around and who is passionate about helping you.*

---

# 5

# What to eat?

I love wine, I love coffee, I love soft cheese, I love entertaining, I love travelling, I love camping, I love celebrating, I love the markets, I love playing sport. All of these things have the enjoyment of easy food. Food is the talk, the planning, the shopping, the preparing, the celebration. It's the endless conversations and messages between family and friends about *What can I bring?*

But seriously, what can I eat whilst trying to get pregnant? What improves my chances of falling pregnant each month? What should I eat? What shouldn't I eat? What foods should I be eating at certain times of the month? Which foods improve my egg count and quality, cycle length, uterus lining, implantation and emotions, and reduce the chance of miscarriage to produce a healthy baby? And which foods help my husband to produce more sperm and sperm that swims faster and is good quality?

What if I drink coffee, soft drink, energy drinks, beer and wine? What if I eat soft cheese, shellfish, raw sushi, deli meats, reheated beef and chicken meals, pâté, raw eggs or pre-packaged salads?

Who do I listen to about what to eat? My doctor, nurses, pharmacist, naturopath, family and friends? Or do I listen to the fertility experts I follow online or have searched on Google, and whose books I have read?

Our social lives mostly revolve around food and drinks. Christmas is all about sitting down to a beautiful meal and eating, Easter is about eating hot cross buns and chocolate eggs, birthdays are about eating cake, picnics in the park are about picnic food, going cycling or to a yoga class is about having a coffee afterwards, celebratory gatherings at work are about morning teas full of sweet spreads, going to the markets is about sampling foods, travelling is about trying different cultural foods and drinks ... hey, just making it through the work week is about celebrating happy hour at 5.00 pm on a Friday.

So much of our lives is around the enjoyment of eating and drinking and in the cooking of new recipes to impress. Then suddenly, it can feel like you really have to look at the foods and drinks you are consuming and question whether they will increase your chances of falling pregnant.

It used to be so easy, just enjoying whatever foods were placed in front of you, but now you really have to think about whether that particular food or drink is suitable for trying to get pregnant.

## THE ALKALINE DIET

My first encounter with foods and drinks for fertility was probably inside a pregnancy magazine. However, this was more directed at women who were already pregnant. I wondered what foods were good for trying to get pregnant. This is when I heard about the alkaline diet. Before this I had never been on a diet or really given much thought as to what I ate or didn't eat. I ate a pretty balanced diet with just a little bit of takeaway food. I had one coffee a day and a couple of drinks each month. I thought all fruits and vegetables were healthy. I never knew anything about food groups, acidic foods, neutral foods or alkaline foods.

Growing up on the farm we mostly ate our own produce, rarely did I have takeaway, lollies or processed foods. The beef, chicken and lamb came from our own farm. I used to open up the freezer and there would be a tongue or liver staring at me. And many of our vegetables were fresh from our farm as well. If we wanted something sweet to eat, we cooked it ourselves from scratch. Cakes, slices, biscuits, desserts. Mum would even make herself Baileys at Christmas. I had never heard of a frozen meal or two-minute noodles until I left home to work in the city.

So when we went to see our first naturopath about trying to fall pregnant, they suggested the alkaline diet. This is where certain foods and fresh produce are good, or bad, for alkalising the body—with the aim being to alkalise the body's pH level. So on the front of our fridge we stuck up a list of the foods in each category.

I found the food list on the fridge annoying; I couldn't quite grasp how a fruit or vegetable could not be beneficial, so I hid the list on the side of the fridge where I couldn't see it.

## THE TRADITIONAL CHINESE WARMING FOODS DIET

Next we went to see the traditional Chinese medicine clinic that was famous for fertility, and this was where our baby making diet got real. This clinic had a very detailed plan for new clients, so much so that we had to do a full-day introduction course on what to eat.

Wow, a full day on Chinese medicine for fertility. I was excited as I thought, *This is it, this is how we have our baby*.

The traditional Chinese medicine diet was all about warming foods and drinks. The warm temperature helps give the body's chi (energy) and blood the strength to conceive and carry a pregnancy through to having a healthy baby. Following a warming diet also helps focus chi and blood circulation on the lower abdomen where the reproductive organs reside—improving blood flow to this area can enhance fertility.

Eating warm stuff to me sounded pretty easy.

As well as warming foods, the clinic also recommended we eat high protein, low carb, low sugar and low-processed foods with warm drinks, such as herbal teas. Out the door went the old toast and cereal for breakfast, and in came eggs, mushrooms, avocado, bacon, cooked tomatoes and baby spinach. Yum, I loved a gourmet breakfast and never really liked sugary boxed cereals to start with. And definitely no drinks from the fridge with ice, so room-temperature water it was. Also, we were advised to drink soy milk instead of cow's milk, so I started buying morning soy lattes instead.

We pretty much followed the Chinese warming diet during the numerous years we were also doing the fertility clinic procedures, including the four IUI cycles and the first four IVF cycles that I did when I was twenty-nine to thirty-one years old.

## THE REPRODUCTIVE VEGGIE DIET

After the years of traditional Chinese medicine high protein, low-carb eating, we had a big break from IVF and just got on with our lives, eating whatever. We still ate reasonably well and kept the white foods down, such as white bread, pasta and potatoes.

One weeknight our friends invited us to join them in the city for a general health information night. There was an American guest speaker talking about how to eat healthy to prevent disease, as they say all disease is preventable. Common diseases such as cancer and arthritis were discussed and the topic of infertility came up as well. I was like a sponge, listening and soaking it all up and taking notes. The speaker advised men to eat fresh figs and asparagus daily as these fruits look like the male reproductive system. Whilst listening to this I had a laugh as I was imagining figs and asparagus in a way I never had before. Oh, and as females we need to eat avocado, pomegranates and stone fruits—the avocado looks like a pregnant belly, and pomegranates have lots of little red seeds inside, just like the female reproductive system. Well, it definitely was an interesting way to look at fruit and vegetables.

At the time I didn't even know what a pomegranate was, let alone know how to put it into my food. And I had never bought figs or asparagus before, but it was kind of fun buying something new.

We gave our reproductive-organ fruit and veggie diet a go for a few months, but got over that pretty quickly. Whenever I think of figs and pomegranates today, I still have a laugh.

## THE BLOOD TYPE DIET

Next, my husband came across the blood type diet. After his two knee surgeries, he had to do a lot of physiotherapy and knee-strengthening exercises to prevent the random shooting knee pain he would get. He also wanted to lose some weight as having less weight on the knee helped. That's how the blood type diet entered our lives.

The principle is to eat beneficial foods based on your blood type, as certain foods will benefit some blood types while the same foods will not benefit other blood types. As my husband and I are both type A, this made life easy as we could buy, prepare and eat the same foods. I think I would have pulled my hair out if we were different blood types as after a long day's work, who really wants to prepare two different meals? Not me!

Similar to the alkaline diet, the blood type diet has three

food categories: beneficial, neutral and avoid. For blood type A we needed to avoid red meat, potatoes, tomatoes, bananas and gluten. It also recommended beneficial types of exercise; for us, we needed to avoid high-impact exercise as our bodies do not respond well to this, and focus instead on general exercise, such as yoga, Pilates, weights, walking and swimming. Yay, I always hated jogging—a sprint was ok but not long-distance running as I felt awkward doing it. And I loved yoga, Pilates and walking.

We did the blood type diet really well and we still roughly follow it now.

## THE TEAS AND PINEAPPLE DIET

We also randomly heard or read about various foods and drinks and if they mentioned the word fertility we would stop and take note. Things like ashwagandha—we bought this and drank it as tea. It is an ancient medicinal herb that has anti-cancer properties, lowers blood sugar levels, reduces stress and anxiety, and can boost testosterone and increase fertility in men. Ok so drink up we did; it's not the most pleasant-tasting drink but we did whatever we could.

I also got stuck into the raspberry leaf tea. Unlike ashwagandha tea, raspberry leaf tea tastes good. And it helps to strengthen the uterine lining and prevent miscarriage.

And then there was pineapple. I read that eating pineapple, including the core, around implantation time increases the chances of conception as it reduces inflammation in the body, including the uterus. Luckily, I like pineapple and still eat heaps of it today, and yes, including the core.

## THE DETOX DIET

One night during our time with Happy Transfer Doctor, when he had arranged another full IVF cycle without listening to my concerns at all, I went onto Google and typed in natural fertility. As you can imagine, heaps of results came up. And up came the 'Seven steps to holistic fertility treatment'. *Wow, that's me,* I thought, *I'm now done with everything else.* I clicked on the link and read everything and it just felt right.

However, I had this little voice in the back of my mind saying, *This expert is based in Ireland and that is the other side of the world ... I'm sure there are other holistic experts in Australia.* Anyway, I just went ahead and emailed Ireland instead. The holistic fertility expert was actually from Australian originally. I emailed her my fertility story and she replied very quickly with a 'Yes, I would love to work with you.' We set up our initial Zoom call. Evening in Australia is morning in Ireland so the timing was great. The first Zoom call was with my husband as well. She recommended that for the next three months we prepare ourselves to be as healthy as possible by following her VIP fertility program, to create the best-possible sperm and eggs for a successful pregnancy.

At first we both had to weigh ourselves and then do a one-week cleanse, which meant no meat, dairy, gluten, sugar, coffee or wine. Wait, did someone say no coffee or wine? How could I possibly survive this? How do you get through the day without a coffee? This was a foreign concept to me and my husband. He was working in the city in a new job at the time, and there were about ten coffee shops on his walk between the train station and his office. And I was working in an office as well, I had my coffee break timed to a tee. Coffee is not just a drink but a lifestyle, or a lifesaver … both, really!

During the initial cleanse we ate vegetable soups, salads, legumes, nuts, whole foods … basically with no animal products. Instead of our morning coffee fix we had dandelion tea, and a green tea at midmorning.

This first week was a real challenge for me, especially not eating any meat. I didn't really eat red meat anyway, but I had been eating a lot of chicken. And I do always need to eat regularly otherwise I feel starving very quickly … hangry, my husband calls it.

The VIP fertility program also involved thirty minutes of exercise every day. So we both kicked into gear with power walking. I would come home from work and change into my exercise clothes and take my dog for a walk every day, and I surprised myself by loving it. Not only was it good exercise but I also really liked the stress relief it provided from being in an office all day. Also, my husband had his long walk to the office and would go out walking during lunch breaks as well.

As a result of all this healthy eating and exercise, we both lost weight. Over the next six months my husband lost seventeen kilograms and I lost six. We also had fortnightly Zoom calls with our naturopath where we would discuss our diet, exercise, emotional health, cycle, work, stress, etc. We basically would aim for a really healthy Monday to Friday and enjoy some coffees and alcoholic drinks on the weekends. This worked really well as most of our socialising was on the weekends.

So when you are on a healthy eating regimen with limited sugar and alcohol, what should you do? Yes, that's right, have a party.

It was a great idea, we had a party at our place where we cooked barbecue foods and a yummy dessert. I had it all worked out, instead of drinking my beloved bottle of red wine I would mix it with a juice to water it down, and remember to drink heaps of water at the same time. So I started off mixing the wine and juice in a mason jar, and I felt pretty cool as everything is cooler in a mason jar! And I was doing so well ... well, up until someone pulled out the tequila.

I have a love/hate relationship with tequila. I really love Mexican food and margaritas, so loving tequila is just a natural progression. However, it does not love me.

But seriously, why is tequila, salt and lemon so good!

Once the tequila came out of the cupboard, I was just going to have half a shot, just one, right? Well, famous last words. Half a shot turned into a whole shot and the downhill slide began.

We had a nice fire going outside and I vaguely remember at one stage, after a few tequilas, lying on the grass next to the fire. And the next minute I was lying on my bathroom floor.

Normally to go to sleep I need the whole house in complete silence with no lights on, even the air conditioner's red power button light in my bedroom is enough to annoy me. And also, many times I have put a pillow against the closed bedroom door to stop the light from coming in underneath. However, after the tequila shots, that night I fell asleep in my bed with the light on, door open and the rest of the party still going on in the house with music, etc. Very surprisingly, the next morning I felt great as I had had a wonderful night's sleep.

So how was I going to answer my naturopath on our next Zoom call when she asked me how my diet was going? *Umm ... well, yes, pretty good except I did have a small gathering at my place and had a couple of drinks.* Well truthfully, the tequila I drank was quickly thrown up afterwards ... this negates me even having any alcohol to start with, right?


So, what are you supposed to eat to help with getting pregnant? The eighty-twenty rule is a good guideline to follow as it removes the pressure of having to eat well with every single mouthful and allows you to relax a little more and enjoy yourself. Eat really well eighty per cent of the time and eat more relaxed twenty per cent of the time. This is in general with food, whether trying to fall pregnant or not.

Or, another way of looking at it is to eat really well Monday to Friday (the eighty per cent) and eat more relaxed on the weekends (the twenty per cent). Usually there are more social outings on the weekends, and this is when you can be more relaxed about what you eat. This goes for coffee and alcohol as well. Avoid them during the week, but enjoy them on the weekends. It's just about being more mindful of what you eat and drink and the quantities.

Also, a note: Stay away from tequila shots, lol!

However, if you have just had an embryo transfer and are in the two-week wait, it's best to avoid all coffee and alcohol. Try herbal tea instead and non-alcoholic wine if you are out and about and feel the need to blend in and drink something from a wine glass.

If you are a coffee lover like I am and the thought of giving up your daily fix is unthinkable, try roasted dandelion coffee. What you resist persists, and I resisted this stuff for so long. I bought a huge bag of it online as I had read great reviews about it on a fertility website and then I didn't drink any for over a year! I was so distraught at the thought of replacing my caffeine fix with this stuff I just couldn't even try it. My husband drank quite a bit of it, but I just couldn't go there. However, when I finally did, OMG, it was so good! My fave is Dandy Blend.

Seek advice from a qualified naturopath who specialises in fertility. And ask them any questions you may have. Following a specialised food plan really helps, especially for couples when you both work.

Follow inspiring healthy foodies on social media. There is nothing like a yummy healthy meal picture to get yourself motivated to get into the kitchen and whip something up. It is also so much more satisfying when you prepare a meal yourself rather than buy a quick fix.

Also, the food channel is amazing for healthy food inspo. Watching someone in a foreign country cooking something healthy in the outdoors is very motivating and it can help you get excited about healthy food.

Another way to get excited about healthy food is to go to your local markets on the weekends. However, instead of just quickly going to the markets and heading home, make a real outing of it. Do a breakfast or brunch or coffee at the markets with your partner or friends. Sit down under a tree and people watch and taste test the food that is on offer.

Invest in the right cooking utensils and equipment for your kitchen. A food processor is a great addition as it can whip up some healthy dips etc. very quickly. We bought one and made a permanent space for it on our kitchen bench as this way we use it more often (instead of having to pull it out of the cupboard). And experiment with new recipes, some will be a flop but it's the joy of trying. I made this very thick mushroom soup once and it looked like a grey sludge, however despite the terrible look, it tasted good.

Listen to your body. Once you start eating healthy you will feel a difference for the better.

# staying sane tips

1. *Adopt the eighty-twenty guideline for healthy eating. Eat really healthy eighty per cent of the time and eat more relaxed the remaining twenty per cent.*

2. *Alternatively, eat really healthy Monday to Friday and eat more relaxed on the weekends. This will help you enjoy your weekends without stressing about what you can and cannot eat when out and about with friends.*

3. *Follow a special fertility eating guideline provided by a naturopath. Having an actual plan with recipes will take any unnecessary stress and guesswork out of what to eat.*

4. *Get inspired by healthy eating bloggers on social media or the food channel on TV. There is nothing like a photo of a yummy healthy meal to get you cooking in the kitchen.*

5. *Make a date with your partner to go to the local farmers' markets. Sample some of the fresh food and get inspired to cook with fresh ingredients.*

6. *Set up your kitchen for big cook-offs. Purchase a food processor and make space on your kitchen bench for it to permanently sit; you will use it more when it is easy to reach.*

7. *Remember that eating healthier will improve your body for baby making, but it will also greatly benefit you in the long term because healthy food is preventative medicine.*

# 6

# Finding your chi

Dear Doctor Google, what can I do naturally to increase my chances of falling pregnant?

Google replies with:

- *7 Ways to Increase Your Odds of Getting Pregnant*

- *Tips for Getting Pregnant - Baby Centre*

- *10 Ways to Boost Your Odds of Getting Pregnant*

- *Ways to Boost Your Fertility*

- *Increase Your Egg Health in 90 Days to Get Pregnant*

- *8 Best Sex Positions to Conceive a Baby*

- *Get Pregnant Faster: Your 7-Step Plan*

- *20 Natural Remedies to Help You Conceive Fast*

For some couples, there comes a time between the fun and excitement of trying to fall pregnant—you're anticipating the day when the pregnancy test kits stashed in your bathroom cupboard show a positive result—and when very suddenly you have thoughts like *Why have I not fallen pregnant yet? How long should it normally take to get pregnant?* and *Is something wrong with me?*

Once these thoughts start it can feel like they are all you ever think about. From quietly joyous, to suddenly worried. How our minds turn so quickly! And this sudden worry takes us to none other than Doctor Google. We madly type into the search field *quick and natural ways to get pregnant*, because we so want to join that mothers group.

And then starts the online researching of ways to get pregnant fast without the dreaded medical intervention. Because you are not on that road just yet. You are in that stage in between "fun and excited" and "how can I speed this thing up already?"

Also, there are the well-meaning friends and family who give you their stories. The ones about themselves or their friends who eat this and that, who saw this person or that naturopath, etc.

*My friend Sarah had been trying to fall pregnant and went to see this great naturopath and fell pregnant straight away.*

*One of the girls at work was struggling to fall pregnant and drank this tea every day for a month and got pregnant.*

*I saw on* A Current Affair *a story about a Chinese doctor who helps people get pregnant.*

With natural therapies, you name it, I have tried it. Anything that I could do naturally without having to go down the medical intervention route I was all in for. As I didn't like needles and wasn't a fan of doctors or hospitals, I really gave natural therapies a decent go.

## BASAL BODY TEMPERATURE CHART

First I read online about a well-known "baby maker" natural clinic and purchased the book that the clinic owner had written. So off we drove, having taken a day off work, and went onto their fertility program. This involved liquid Chinese herbs and basal body temperature charting. So I bought myself a thermometer and every morning when I woke up I took my temperature under my tongue and recorded it on the printed chart I had been given.

During the middle of a cycle your temperature should chart slightly lower before ovulation and slightly higher just after ovulation due to the increased amounts of progesterone. This should reveal two distinct phases in your graph, therefore indicating your best time to conceive. However, each body is different, so it is recommended that you chart several cycles to understand the specific way you experience the basal body temperature cycle.

I would complete each month's chart and email it through to the clinic. They would interpret it and send more herbs to drink depending on my specific chart for the following month. The temperature charting didn't really show me any significant changes throughout my cycle. We tried this for a while, but nothing happened, so we didn't continue with it. I felt disheartened that my temperature chart didn't provide me with much clarity on when I was most fertile.

## CHINESE HERBS

The next stop on my natural therapies journey was at the big one, the Chinese medicine man. This clinic had a very well-known fertility program. I saw a story about the clinic on TV that showed lots of successful babies and I was super excited when making the initial phone call to the clinic the very next day. As mentioned in Chapter 5, to join their fertility program we had to attend a mandatory full-day information session at the clinic where we learnt all about the program—from Chinese yin and yang theory, to diet, stress management, emotional health, Chinese medicine, acupuncture and exercise.

A large part of Chinese medicine is chi, which means aliveness or life-force energy. According to traditional Chinese medicine, the body has natural patterns of chi that circulate throughout the body via the meridian channels. When certain meridians are out, so is the chi linked to that meridian's organ/s, therefore disrupting the energy flow. Acupuncture, diet and reducing stress helps improve the life-force energy and the organ meridians.

The initial Chinese medicine we tried was fresh herbs. So out came the cooking pot and in went the dried herbs, which looked like the result of a bushwalk where I had just gone and picked up leaves, dirt and stuff from the ground. So you just put the twigs into a pot with water and simmer them on the stove. Once they have cooled, bottoms up, you drink it.

The herbs smelt and tasted pretty bad. But you know I really wanted that baby, so I would drink the twigs like a fine wine, or more like tequila—I would throw that crap back and hopefully not bring it back up. But, unlike with tequila, I didn't want to dance on tables afterwards, instead I had a big glass of water ready to skull straight after drinking the herbs to take away the lingering twig taste.

After the fresh herbs, we graduated to tablet herbs and supplements, which were so much better. No more cooking twigs over the stove, just tablets from a bottle.

I had to take the Chinese herbs and supplements at specific times during my monthly cycle and the clinic would send me a new batch every fortnight depending on my cycle symptoms. Therefore, I had to call them on the first day of my cycle, and again on day fifteen. During these calls they would ask me numerous questions such as what day of my cycle was I on, what colour was the discharge, how was the flow, were there any clots, how was I feeling, what were my energy levels, etc. However, making these regular calls was a bit challenging as the clinic was only open during business hours and I also worked business hours. I did have a telephone at my desk, but how could I talk about my period when there were colleagues within earshot? *Yes, I'm on day one, the colour is nice and red, I'm feeling ok.* Hmm, no, I didn't make these calls from my desk, instead I would grab my mobile and walk outside. However, just outside there are heaps of windows looking back into all the offices. So every two weeks I would walk well into the work car park and talk about my cycle flow, surrounded by cars. Then the clinic would post the Chinese herbs I would take for the next two weeks, and where did they post them? Yes, you guessed it, I got them posted to work as I wasn't at home during the week to sign for the courier and I'm sure the reception girls all read the sender details and knew what I was receiving.

I wasn't the only one doing the Chinese herbs and supplements, my husband also did. However, his were different to mine and they weren't timed as per my cycle.

Our relationship with this clinic stayed strong all through when we were trying to fall pregnant naturally, then the four IUI procedures, and into the start of our IVF journey for four embryo transfers. It was very helpful to call and speak with the clinic, especially when I started doing IVF, as it was great to get tips on what I could also be doing to increase my chances and also just to talk procedures, herbs, medications or anything that was on my mind with someone to get another perspective on things. It was like I had my very own team cheering me on.

## ACUPUNCTURE

To complement the Chinese medicine herbs and supplements, this clinic also offered acupuncture as part of the protocol.

I had never had acupuncture before. Hmm, I didn't even like needles, so how was I going to go a whole bunch of small needles all over my body, including my head? Well, funny what wanting a baby will do to you. I booked myself in to see the acupuncturist and got needled. I made sure I had the most experienced acupuncturist as I didn't want a work experience kid. And to my surprise, these little needles do not hurt, and it was nothing like a blood test. At first the needle twinges for about half a second and then you can't feel it at all.

I found the acupuncture to be relaxing and helpful, like I could sense my meridians aligning.

My acupuncture sessions were timed as per my monthly cycle dates. My husband also did acupuncture, but he just did regular fortnightly sessions.

It was a challenge at first to go to the regular acupuncture appointments on the other side of the city on weekdays when we both worked. However, shortly after starting their fertility program, our clinic advised that they had a new acupuncturist working from our very own suburb. Wow, this was such a huge relief as it just made attending appointments so much easier.

So began our adventure with this local acupuncturist. We would see her fortnightly. If she moved premises, we would follow. I heard all about her kids, husband, other clients, marriage breakdown, divorce, etc. Yes, she was an over sharer, but what can you do but listen when you have a heap of needles stuck in your body, and sometimes a heat lamp or moxa box burning over your belly?

Thoughts used to cross my mind like what if I suddenly sneezed … would I hit the heat lamp that was hovering just above my belly and burn myself? You know, things you think about when trying to relax. But when that crazy thought left my mind I would use this time to relax, focus on my breathing, visualise a baby growing inside and think of baby names. Other times I would just pray, *Please please please please please let me be pregnant.*

## HYPNOTHERAPY

Another thing I tried was hypnotherapy. One of my friends had recently been to see a hypnotherapist and I thought, why not! I looked up the hypnotherapist's website and she helped people stop smoking, lose weight, and get the confidence to change their lives. Well, I was in. So I booked myself in just before I decided to do my first IVF cycle, as I was stressing about the needles and the whole process in general.

Off I drove one day, again another work day that I had taken off. I headed up the coast for the one-hour drive. When I walked into the clinic, I felt relaxed; the hypnotherapist had a lovely, calming presence. I sat down in the big, comfy hypno chair. And I started the hypnotherapy session. I wanted to work on my fear of needles and the whole medical intervention thing … doctors and hospitals, etc.

Now, this hypnotherapy is definitely not like the crazy performances you see in cringe-worthy comedy lounges. It is more like a one-on-one therapy session. I advised the hypnotherapist about my fears and we got to work. Before we started, she asked for my permission to record our session and she would upload my recording so that I could do it at home. I closed my eyes and we started, I basically repeated what she said.

Now I never went into a full trance or anything, I remembered it all. And when the session finished, I felt relaxed and more positive about needles, doctors and hospitals, like it had taken the edge off.

I did go back to see the hypnotherapist for one more session, but I was never totally cured. Maybe I would have been if I went to more sessions.

Five years later when I went back and did another full cycle of IVF after having a break for a number of years, I bought an online hypnotherapy for fertility program. This was easy as I just uploaded it to my iPod and would listen to it each night when I was going to sleep. Each recording was a quick ten minutes and I enjoyed this and found it to be very beneficial for getting to sleep.

## YOGA

I have always enjoyed yoga and Pilates and I used to do them as a form of easy exercise at home to stretch out my shoulders and back from sitting at a desk all day. I definitely didn't do it as a form of relaxation, mindfulness or stress relief. So one day when I came across a program called Yoga for Fertility, I was sold … again. I had not heard of doing yoga for specific health concerns. However, there are certain yoga positions you can do to help with falling pregnant. I was so excited by this as I could work on my body and fall pregnant as well … winner!

## MEDITATION

I had read and heard so much about meditation and the amazing results, however had never tried it as the thought of sitting still and focusing on my breath seemed hard—my brain was always racing ahead of me. One of my friends had opened up a massage therapy clinic and started a weekly meditation evening. So off I went to meditation on a weeknight, as I thought I had to give it a proper professional try.

We all sat cross legged on the floor with cushions, closed our eyes, smelt the burning essential oils and relaxed. We did guided meditations, so would listen and follow in our minds. Sometimes we would follow a rainbow.

However, at the end of one hour sitting crossed legged, everything was numb. I was so uncomfortable and was peeking out of one eye around the room to see if anyone else was sitting in pain. Nope, they all had seen the rainbow.

Afterwards we would open our eyes and go around the room talking about what we had seen and felt. *Ummm, I can't feel my lower body*, I wanted to say. The others had such great meditations, but I struggled to see or feel anything.

However, I did go back and do this weekly for a while, but instead of sitting crossed legged I would lie on the floor, which was so much better.

Only very recently I have given meditation another go. Instead of the one-hour sessions, I just do five to ten minutes at home where I'm in a more relaxed environment and not trying to compare myself to the others in the room. And surprisingly, I have really enjoyed it. Also, meditation does not happen instantly, as I used to think, instead it is a practice and therefore you can do little bits often.

## KINESIOLOGY

Another thing I got into was kinesiology. At first I thought it was similar to acupuncture but without the actual needles. I soon learnt that there was so much more to it. Kinesiology is where the practitioner does muscle testing to identify imbalances within the body and the meridians.

I got so sucked into this "new thing" that instead of just going to see a kinesiologist, I ended up joining a school to study kinesiology. Before I knew it I was going to a full weekend course once a month. This all happened very quickly as the yearly course intake was starting that same month.

The first couple of weekend studies were really interesting, I even held a study day at my house with some of the students one Saturday, and other times I went to another student's house. However, by the fourth weekend I was way in over my head with also working full time and I quit. I think I had just been trying to find a new hobby to get into, but I now realise that the study of kinesiology is very full on and you really have to be one hundred per cent committed to it.

However, during my short-lived studies I met one student who I still see for kinesiology balances today. So instead of studying kinesiology, I go to a session and get myself balanced instead.

The thing I love about kinesiology is that it realigns your body physically but it is also like a therapy session because it clears any mental or emotional blocks you may have. I found it so beneficial when I was going through the keyhole surgery and IVF cycles.

## HOMEOPATHY

As mentioned in Chapter 5, when we were on the detox diet with the naturopath in Ireland, I also tried homeopathic remedies for the first time. On our fortnightly Zoom calls I was asked about diet and stress, and also about my cycle, and from this information I was mailed homeopathic tablets.

Homeopathy is a system of natural health care that treats each person as an individual by stimulating their own healing ability.

So in the mail arrived this envelope with little white tablets inside that I would take on various days of my cycle. I would just put them under my tongue and they would dissolve ... easy.

After my first month of being on the little white tablets and detoxing and exercising every day, I felt wonderful. My next period arrived and there were no symptoms leading up to it and no pain or discomfort at all, which was so strange for me. (Even when I had been on the full Chinese medicine program, I still experienced pain every month.) And it also helped my digestion, so I was completely sold on homeopathy; these teeny tiny tablets had a huge impact.

## EMOTIONAL FREEDOM TECHNIQUE

During calls with my naturopath in Ireland, we would also discuss my emotional health to see if I had any emotional blocks coming up. And with the ups and downs of infertility, I definitely had some.

I was advised to do emotional freedom technique tapping,

otherwise known as EFT tapping. I had heard of it and yes, was willing to give anything a go.

I found EFT tapping to be quick and effective, especially with the everyday demands of work, exercise, preparing healthy meals and going to an array of appointments, from doctor visits to acupuncture and kinesiology sessions. I would watch an EFT video on YouTube and tap for about eight minutes before bed, and I still do this for various reasons today. It just feels nice, it makes you stop for a moment and focus on one thing—that being your own self-care.

## SUPPLEMENTS

Next on the list with the Ireland naturopath was vitamin supplements. There was a supplement company in the UK that specifically did a high-end fertility package for both men and women. The ingredient dosages were much higher and she had had very good results from this supplement company. The only thing was, they don't sell these supplements in Australia. However, we could order them on their UK website and they would ship them to Australia.

First of all, the fertility package was expensive. Fertility is kind of like weddings, when you say it is for fertility, the price just jumps right up. When I converted the supplements into AUD and applied the shipping cost I nearly fainted. Could we afford this? Well, as we had already invested in the VIP fertility program, we thought we may as well go the full hog. I clicked "order" on their website.

A week later, we received an email from the Australian customs; they wanted to know what supplements we were trying to bring into the country. They wanted the full ingredient list of each bottle, and there were heaps of bottles. So we emailed the supplement company and requested this, and forwarded it to customs. A few days later we receive our many glass bottles of supplements in a big box.

We ended up placing another order of these supplement packages and boy were we healthy. It was like we were oozing good vitamins out of our pores.

## FENG SHUI

Another thing I read about was feng shui. This is a Chinese system of laws that believes the spatial arrangement and orientation of furniture has an effect on the flow of energy (chi) in the home. In other words, there are favourable or unfavourable effects depending on the furniture arrangements. *Feng* means wind and *shui* means water. I thought this was pretty interesting and read up on feng shui, which resulted in a total rearrangement of our master bedroom. I moved the bedhead from one wall to the opposite wall. I'm not sure if I felt any energy flow change from this, but I think mentally I felt better just knowing that the feng shui was improved.

At the end of the day, you need to do what feels good to you. Use your intuition; if you get a good gut feeling about a natural therapy, research it then give it a go. Don't regret any of the natural therapies you have used that may not have given you that baby, because that therapy has most likely given you other tools to use for life. I now regularly go to acupuncture, take homeopathic tablets and eat healthy, practise yoga and EFT tapping, and have just started to do my own little meditations at home. And I'm doing these for myself and not for anyone else or anything other than my own self-care.

Try to keep doing a natural therapy that makes you feel better afterwards. One that makes you feel light, positive and in control of your emotions, and is helpful on your baby-making train ride. When I would drive the forty-five minutes to see my kinesiologist, I would be feeling scatterbrained and like I was all over the place, however on the drive home it was as if I were a new person. My mind would be clearer and I felt so positive. It was the same with the acupuncture, the time lying on the bed with the needles doing their thing forced me to stop and relax. And on leaving those many appointments I felt so much stronger.

Ask the natural therapist what their follow-up service is, as you will get so much more from that relationship if they follow up afterwards to see how you are going; even if the follow-up is just by email, this will keep things moving along in a positive way for you. It will help keep your practice front of your mind and help you remove any blocks that may have come up in between your appointments.

It can be so helpful when you go to an appointment and sometimes just talk to your natural therapist about anything that comes to mind. In comparison to talking with a good friend or family member, a natural therapist can give you so many tools when you are on this emotional roller-coaster. They understand the fertility process and all the effects of the medication if you are doing IVF, etc. So really let them know what is on your mind; even if you think it's nothing, it probably is something that they can assist with.

Also include your partner or husband on the natural therapy journey, as they are experiencing a similar emotional roller-coaster as well. And they may have other things that come up for them. If you are paying for a fertility program, include them as much as possible; it will be so helpful for them and will also bring you closer as you can really open up and share the experience.

Sometimes you might have "shining new object syndrome" where you are currently seeing one natural therapist and you hear or read about another type of natural therapy that could be better. You know when you hear or read about another therapy and you are so tempted to include that as well. Maybe this new therapy will get you what you want. However, as there are so many things going on in your life when you are on the baby making train, it is best to focus on one natural therapy fertility program at a time. Just try not to overfill your plate as it might be too much for your body and mind to focus on.

In regards to relaxation techniques such as meditation, hypnotherapy and EFT tapping, if at first you don't think you are switching off quick enough or if you go to a class and think you may not be getting enlightened like the other people in the class, but if it does feel like you are taking one teeny tiny step in the right direction, keep at it. Any kind of time out from the baby-making train ride, and time out from your brain working overtime going over all the *What if?* scenarios, is a step on the path to emotional freedom.

There is absolutely no harm in having more relaxation, more mind/body connection, , more healthy foods, more chi flowing through your body from the Chinese herbs, or a clearer mind from the hypnotherapy. Nor is there harm in light exercise, releasing any type of emotional block by EFT tapping or kinesiology, or creating a more flowing home from good feng shui.

# staying sane tips

1. *Trust your intuition, do your research. If a natural therapy feels good, give it a go.*

2. *Keep your chosen natural therapy program relevant in your life with follow-up service between appointments. This will release any small emotional blocks that might have come up quickly.*

3. *Be completely open and honest with your natural therapist, as they have so much experience in the fertility field and extensive knowledge of IVF medication effects, etc.*

4. *Include your partner or spouse with the natural therapy, if you have one, as they too are experiencing emotions and it will also bring you closer as a couple.*

5. *Stay focused on one natural therapy fertility program at a time so that you don't get overwhelmed with too much on your plate.*

6. *If you can't switch off when doing meditation, hypnotherapy or EFT tapping, just remember that you are getting a good relax in, so stick with it. They are a practice and with practise they become easier and more potent.*

YouTube has many EFT tapping videos for fertility, making it so quick and easy to release any emotional blocks.

# 7

# Fifty shades of ... ovulation kits and temperature charts

Sex—When you are young, it is so spontaneous

Sex—When you are trying to have a baby, it is hopeful, lighthearted and fun

Sex—When you have been trying to have a baby for a while, it gets a little less glamorous and a lot more stressful

Sex—After you have been trying to have a baby for ages, it gets to be a thing on your to-do list and worry settles in

Sex—When you are on IVF drugs and Chinese herbs, it is all pre-scheduled by the timing

When you are seriously trying for a baby and it hasn't happened yet, there are so many things that can go through your mind. When it is that time to get down and dirty, instead of nice romantic thoughts you may be thinking:

Beforehand: Is the timing right tonight? Am I ovulating? Am I stressed today? Did I have time to do meditation today?

During: Is this position best for conceiving? Was the ovulation test result just a faint line or a dark line? The Chinese medicine therapist said we both have to orgasm to conceive, is this going to happen tonight? Did I put the dishwasher on?

After: Have we finally just made a baby? Do I need to prop my belly up with a heap of pillows and stay laying down? Or should I put my legs in the air? Oh no, I need to sneeze!

As mentioned in Chapter 6, when we went to our first natural therapy clinic, they recommended I do basal body temperature charting to check if there was a pattern for my ovulation. On my temperature chart that I needed to complete each morning, I also had to record what days we had sex by putting a little circle around the date.

It felt really weird circling the days we had sex on a piece of paper and emailing this to a stranger. It was very clinical, like a compulsory assignment you had to hand in and get graded on, with the anticipation of hopefully getting an A+. And I double checked to make sure I was only emailing the clinic and not all the contacts in my email account!

I stopped recording my temperature when I bought the jumbo pack of ovulation kits from China, as these were so much simpler. I just had to pee on a stick a few times during the middle of the month, rather than take my temperature every morning. And then it was just timing serious baby-making sex around ovulation. Other times sex would be just for fun. This was actually quite good as I wasn't stressing about timing and taking my temperature all month long.

When we decided to get serious and went to see the Chinese medicine man to combine Chinese herbs, acupuncture and a warming foods diet, as mentioned in Chapter 6, our previous knowledge of having serious baby making sex only on ovulation days went out the window.

During the information session at the Chinese medicine clinic, a big topic that was covered was sex and how often we were to have it. In Chinese medicine they believe that you can fall pregnant on any day during a monthly cycle. I remember a story the natural therapist told about a couple where the husband was in the defence force and was only home for one weekend and the wife fell pregnant. However, that particular weekend her cycle day wasn't in the normal fertile window, it was at the very end of her cycle but she still fell pregnant. Therefore the natural therapist said that pregnancy can happen on any day of the month, as everyone is different.

Our therapist told all the couples in the room during this information scssion that we had to do "it" every second day. Wow, every second day! We weren't in our honeymoon phase anymore! We were a busy working couple having to battle traffic every day, trying to exercise every day, trying to eat healthy every day, trying to relax every day. Now we had to schedule in sex every second day!

Oh well, I kind of thought that sex was good exercise so I figured it would be my form of exercise for that day. Tick that box, right!

And as it was every second night, it took the guessing game out. It wasn't like one of us would be up for it and the other had a headache. If we really wanted to pin our baby photo up on the wall of the clinic as heaps of other successful couples had done, we had to get on with it every second night as that was part of the program we were paying for.

When we went to the evening information session about healthy eating and the reproductive veggie diet, the advice for trying to get pregnant also went to what positions were ideal. And it was revealed that doggie style was the most beneficial for conception. Hmm, it wasn't on the top of my list. And also, it was recommended that after baby making the female lay on her belly, with pillows under her waistline, whilst also visualising the sperm meeting the egg and conceiving a baby. I did try this visualisation, but I was getting a bit disheartened. By this stage I had done a number of natural therapies, IUIs, and IVF cycles. I wondered, after all the treatments I'd been through, was propping my belly up with pillows after sex and visualising conceiving a baby really going to do anything?

And when you start talking about sex, why not talk about orgasms as well, since we are all friends here! As mentioned, we had both been advised that orgasms were required to conceive. No pressure, right? I was were even told to have an orgasm in the morning right before we had an embryo transfer during an IVF cycle, as it helps the uterus prepare for conception. So again we had timed sex before driving into the city for transfers. My schedule was full.

With all this baby-making sex, sometimes you may need a little help. Bring in the lubricant. I didn't really think much of it until one time I was online reading a baby-making blog and an ad on the side of the page popped up: *Pre-seed: the sperm friendly lubricant that mimics a female's own fertile fluids.* Ok, something else I had never thought of. I was soon madly typing at the keyboard, going into overdrive doing research. (Good thing I did this research on my home computer and not at work on a lunch break!)

Who knew that lubricants were full of chemicals that can kill off good sperm? Commercial lubricants negatively affect sperm motility, making it harder for the sperm to reach the egg. So I quickly bought some Pre-Seed, as the alternatives from my online research were stuff from the pantry. I wasn't that keen on using cooking ingredients such as olive oil, vegetable oil or even egg whites! Apparently they are safe and effective to use, but not what I had in mind.

The funny thing about Pre-Seed is that you have to prepare yourself for sex about ten minutes prior by inserting it in the vagina. And this was supposed to be timed around your most fertile time, as it wasn't the cheapest stuff. So again, to get down to serious baby making, we had to not only schedule it in but also pre-plan the lubricant.

With all this serious baby making, timed days of the month, strategic positions and sperm-friendly lubrication, how do you keep the romance, connection and fun with your partner?

Have exciting things to look forward to together, such as mini vacays. Book in weekends away, long holidays, camping trips, etc. Book a hotel night in the city or coast for your wedding anniversary. There are so many accommodation websites that offer great deals. The best investment is in your relationship and self-love.

Even if you can't always do nights away, plan day trips such as a drive through to the mountains for a hike or coffee; drive on the beach in a four-wheel drive and set up a gazebo for a day of swimming and relaxing, or explore a new farmers' market and eat some yummy healthy food.

If you are using ovulation kits or temperature charts to plan your serious baby making sex, remember that there are all the other times of the month when sex can be just for fun. The benefit of ovulation kits and temperature charts is that there's no need to stress about baby making all month long.

If you're worried that having sex every second day is adding to your already full to-do list, just think of sex as good exercise that relieves stress and releases endorphins. And hey, you don't need expensive activewear to do this type of exercise!

Remember to keep a balance between the serious baby making sex and the just-for-fun sex. If your mind starts taking over, try to turn the mental chatter off. Bring your mind back to the present moment. Say to yourself, *I'm not going to think and worry about our future with or without a baby, I'm going to enjoy this moment right now.* Slowly take six big, deep breaths. Also, there are heaps of meditations online specifically for fertility, download a few of these to have on hand when you feel your mind chatter is taking over.

If your mind keeps wandering off to the stress of the

unknown future, you can even try the elastic band trick. Wear an elastic band on your wrist and when you catch yourself stressing about the future, snap the elastic band to remind yourself to come back to the present moment. Even if you are in the middle of the tango, snap that band if you need to! This sounds silly but it really does help to bring yourself back to the now. I'd often be at home watching a movie and when my mind wandered off to stressing about the unknown future, you could hear me going 'Ouch!'

Think about your partner and the connection that you have, that special something that only you two share. Focus on your connection and have fun together. This doesn't always have to be about the actual sex. Be silly with each other. Play some loud music and dance around the kitchen like a dork. The sillier the dance moves, the funnier they are. Try the boneless chicken dance: *Ok Google, "boneless chicken dance,* The Graham Norton Show"*. This one is so silly you cannot help but crack up laughing with each other.

A good laugh together every day is a must as it makes you smile and brings back that lightness and your inner fun self that can easily get buried beneath the serious baby-making stress.

When you bring in that lightness and fun, this will also help remove the high expectations and judgement around serious baby making. If your mind is only on serious baby-making sex and not on lightness and fun sex, it is so easy to get into the high-expectation mindset, where you are expecting your partner to only produce the best sperm and expecting that your own body cycle is at its most fertile time. When you have such high expectations, you are putting unnecessary stress and pressure on yourself and your partner. Go with the mindset of no expectations, as when you remove the high expectations, you might be pleasantly surprised. And isn't it nice to be happily surprised in life from time to time?

# staying sane tips

1. *Don't get overwhelmed by the regular baby making sex, think of it as exercise that decreases stress and increases good endorphins.*

2. *Book fun weekends away or day trips where you can focus on your connection with your partner.*

3. *Turn off the negative mind chatter by wearing an elastic band on your wrist and snapping it if you catch yourself in a negative mindset. This will bring you back to the present.*

4. *Focus on the special connection that only you have with your partner.*

5. *Remember to include lightness and fun by having a good laugh together every day. Dance around the kitchen like a dork or watch funny cat videos and laugh together.*

6. *Remove the high expectation placed on your partner to perform and your own body to conceive. Go with no expectations and you might be pleasantly surprised.*

7. *You are in it together, so look after each other and have open communication.*

# 8

# Making money to make a baby

If you are trying to fall pregnant but struggling, going down the IVF, acupuncture, supplements and natural therapies route is going to get expensive. I can tell you this from experience. It is not just like going to a GP once for a sickness. A lot of money can be forked out for that little bundle of joy, with hope as the only guarantee and whether you can live with that choice on how much to fork out.

When you walk past the newsagency, you often see on the front pages of the trash magazines pictures of older celebrities with baby bumps—Didn't they just break up with someone last week? And this week they are glowing with a baby bump? And aren't they over thirty-five years old?—or gorgeous newborn babies, but the celebrity was not carrying the baby themselves. Sarah Jessica Parker, Nicole Kidman, Tyra Banks, Kim Kardashian and Elizabeth Banks all had babies via surrogacy.

IVF is expensive! A few cycles to start with is manageable, but it does start getting pretty expensive the more rounds you do. And each year it seems like the medical rebates get lower and lower. It isn't just the IVF; there is the hospital excess for the egg pick-up procedure, the anaesthetist, days off work for yourself and your partner, acupuncture, Chinese herbs, supplements, progesterone gel and the list goes on.

Australian IVF costs are very comparable to the rest of the world. There are cheaper countries such as India, but they are much riskier and have a higher potential for things to go wrong.

The cost of Australian surrogacy can be more expensive; it is about three times more than a regular IVF cycle, as there are no medical rebates. Also, as mentioned in Chapter 4, only certain clinics will do surrogacy IVF as many of the saint-name hospital clinics will not due to religious issues. And there's the fact that in Australia the birth mother is the rightful mother and listed on the birth certificate, not the intended mother who used her own biological eggs, so there are the many legal and financial implications of adoption to think about.

At first, we had money to burn as we had saved up a deposit for our first home, which was before the housing boom, and both worked full time and didn't spend much money on things. We were definitely not thinking about saving for retirement or long-term career goals. It was just the present and in the present we wanted a family. Spending money on natural therapies for fertility was easy. Don't get me wrong, it does add up, but I never wanted to add it up, I just felt it was needed and we could afford it.

When the natural therapies were not producing that baby, we upgraded to private health insurance as there was a twelve-month waiting period and in the back of my mind I felt we needed this insurance to assure IVF if we decided to do it. I was crossing fingers, toes, everything, as I really hated needles and hospitals, but knowing that I had private health insurance did set my mind at ease ... well, to some degree.

And when the first cycle of IVF came around, my professionally organised corporate worker self went into overdrive and I kept all the paperwork and receipts in a nicely sorted plastic sleeve folder (which I still have today). I would walk into Medicare and get my refunds and yes, keep those receipts as well.

Our first year of IVF, when we did three full cycles and one frozen cycle, we had the "baby" money just sitting in our mortgage account. So I didn't worry about money, I only really worried about the needles, operations and falling pregnant. We were lucky we didn't have this extra worry.

Yes, when each cycle didn't work I would "balance the account" and see how many thousands we had just gone through with no baby to show for it. However, we were young and healthy and we still had money and time on our side.

How quickly that feeling of financial security can change. Then came our "anything goes" year off from IVF, with my husband getting a new job in the mines and us travelling to Canada for a white Christmas ... And my husband attempting to ski like he an Olympian and fracturing his knee at Whistler on his first run down the mountain.

Suddenly we had to think about jobs and finances. All that paid sick leave my husband had had at his previous job was gone and he couldn't go back to his new fly-in fly-out job. This was when he decided to go back to university to study a postgraduate degree at the same time as trying to fix his knee with physio, acupuncture and exercises, which all added up to more money. So he studied, worked casually, and tried to fix his knee.

Eleven months after the skiing accident, he was booked in for keyhole surgery and had to have two weeks completely off walking and driving. If he could not drive, he also could not work, so again our easy days of no money concerns were getting a bit old. We had to think about money.

However, after the keyhole surgery, Christmas break and a lot of cold emails to prospective employers, he got a two-days-a-week job in his new chosen field, which he did not have any experience in. So he started there in about March, however that bloody knee was not magically healing as we had hoped it would. Thankfully his job turned into full time by June. However, another operation was looming. This operation was the next best thing to a full knee replacement. No more keyhole stuff—this was a full cut down the front of the knee and six weeks at home with no driving. He had only been at his new job for a few months so there wasn't much paid sick leave.

Another issue we had was that both our cars were manual transmission and because my husband had broken his left knee, he couldn't operate the clutch. He was cleared to drive an automatic car after four weeks, so we decided to sell one of our manual cars and bought an automatic car. He was then able to drive to the office and take the elevator to his desk job.

Funny how an accident can change the course of your life. I thought after the second knee operation that his knee would magically be brand new again. But no, it took another six to twelve months of exercises and physio. To this day he has to make sure that he regularly exercises his knee as when he stops, it seizes up.

After his knee had its time to heal from the second operation, life settled down into a normal flow. And as we didn't want to go through the unexpected and unplanned financial downturn again, we thought we would get ahead through property investment. Yes, it was a risk, but the numbers looked great and we trusted the sales spiel from the property development manager. But we had never built any houses before or dealt with tenants, accountants, lawyers, councils or town planners. And we didn't do much due diligence of our own on the projected figures or the property development manager himself as we should have. But that didn't stop us, and we signed the dotted line. However, the promise from our property development manager of a 13–18 month project timeframe turned into a number of years, and we sacked him a year and a half into the project and ended up doing it ourselves.

Along with the stresses of having no idea what we were doing with this property development project, just that a lot of money was going out, there was a downturn in the resource industry that my husband worked in and he was slowly made redundant—slowly by way of being reduced to four days a week, then three days, etc. However, he picked up some work with his old boss doing garden landscaping.

During this time, we also invited our teenage niece to move in with us as she was studying and wanted to travel overseas when she finished. We had a spare room and it would help her save up for her travels. This was a bit of an eye opener for me as I saw what teenagers spend money on, things like expensive luxury items, which was a lot different from when I was that age.

My husband has had a few different careers and always seems to land on his feet … that is, until he falls off his feet literally. A few months working full time as a landscape gardener and with his boss being overseas for work, my husband was flat out with a number of massive jobs and had a few other guys working with him. One day he was using an electric hedge trimmer while standing on a retaining wall only half a metre above the ground when he tripped over his own feet and fell to the ground. In the process of falling, he threw the trimmer into the garden in front of him, thankfully, otherwise the hedger may have come down with him and cut off a limb. He broke his collarbone and was taken to hospital. However, at the hospital the doctor discovered that he had also fractured his neck. Now this wasn't the first time he had fractured his neck! Previously he had fractured it bodyboarding in the surf when he was a teenager.

So now he was off work again! This time for three months and no driving at all. He did get paid this time, but workers' compensation only pays up to seventy-five per cent of a wage as incentive for the injured person to get back to work as soon as possible.

These things always seem to happen at the worst time, with my husband's boss being overseas and the business being very busy, with my husband the main go-to guy. Also my work was crazy busy and we had our niece living with us trying to organise her end-of-year exams. And the lovely property development pain-in-the-butt issue was still pressing.

During the three months of recovery when I was working, grocery shopping, cooking, cleaning and doing all of the driving, I was actually thankful that I didn't have a small child to look after as well. My husband did try to do stuff around the house as soon as he could, such as cook and vacuum with one arm. My longing for a child completely went out the door. But wait, I had gone through infertility and had embryos in the freezer, wasn't I still desperate for a child?

I then felt guilty for my thankfulness that I didn't have a child, especially with all the things that I had done to try to have one. I remember driving home from work one day knowing that my husband and niece would be at home, and I had this thought: *If I discovered that I was pregnant, how would I feel?* And the answer was that I would be shit scared. I had so longed for that excited feeling of discovering that I was pregnant, but now that I was a bit older and had gone through many challenges, would I be happy to discover I was pregnant? In that moment, the answer was no.

There had been so many perfect times in the past for a pregnancy, when we were younger and had more time, energy and money. However, at thirty-eight years old, when all these challenges were going down, I totally lost my excitement for a pregnancy and baby. This was a strange feeling and I think I tried to ignore it for a while. I just focused on my husband getting better and getting back to work. And helping our niece get sorted for her overseas working holiday.

About six months after my husband returned to work, when our niece had just left for overseas, a close family friend rang to offer us something unbelievable ... they offered to carry our baby for us. Wow, this was totally out of the blue and such a surprise that we didn't know what to think for the next day. I knew that surrogacy was way more expensive than regular IVF; even though we had the frozen embryos it was still, like, brand-new-SUV vehicle expensive and we didn't have the spare cash readily available for it. And there were no guarantees that the embryo would stick first go. I was very surprised and completely grateful to this person for thinking about us in such a generous and loving way.

By the following day when I was driving home, as I seem to do a lot of thinking about life when I drive, I thought ... *Ok, so this might be how we have our baby. We might even get a nice article written up in the* New Idea *magazine about it* ... even though I had no idea if it would work the first time or how we were going to pay for it.

But just when I had recovered from the initial shock and surprise and had come around to the idea that maybe this is how we have our baby, this generous offer was retracted.

I must admit I had slightly got my hopes up for one day, just a little, as I knew deep down we could not afford the surrogacy without going into debt, especially when there were no guarantees it would work. If only we were rich celebrities! But still, that moment of excitement was there one day and gone the next. However, I was so used to hopes rising and being dashed from my years of IVF that I just carried on.

Now that things are going really well and life has settled down, my husband is back at work at full capacity, even going to boot camp classes. Our niece is enjoying her overseas working holiday. My work is going well and we have been on numerous mini holidays. I still haven't got that feeling of desperately wanting a baby back. And I honestly don't think I will. And has money played a part in my thoughts on this? Absolutely. If I didn't have the embryos in the freezer I would have closed this baby door completely, however it is still slightly ajar because every six months I get the bill in the mail to pay the embryo storage fees.

Also, if we had not tried to "get ahead" in our finances by doing the property development that we started when I was thirty-five, we would have still had the spare cash to do the frozen embryo transfers and maybe one or two out of these five could have been little humans by now. However, we will never know now.

I think now that my husband and I have turned forty, we are not so young anymore. Yes, we eat well and exercise, but we cannot turn that number back … we still tick that age bracket box on the forms that says forty plus. Also, before turning forty we didn't really think much about getting older or retirement savings. Now it is something that is thought of and talked about more. In the past we would have easily dropped thousands of dollars on IVF without a second thought, now I think of all the other things I could put those thousands to. If we were *guaranteed* a baby with that money, ok yes, sign me up, but now it is only a very small chance that after forking the money out a healthy, bouncing baby will arrive.

It is a hard realisation that money has to come into many couple's minds when trying to have a baby. If couples have to go the full IVF clinic route, they do have to think about if they can afford it, as it would be an extra challenge starting a pregnancy and giving birth in debt from medical bills.

However, there are many new low-cost IVF clinics in Australia now. These clinics are recommended more for low-complication IVF patients, so if you are starting out, are under forty years old and don't have any major health issues, definitely research them. The costs can be so much cheaper than traditional IVF clinics. They keep the costs down by having the patient appointments with nurses instead of doctors. Fewer medications and stimulation injections are administered, so there's a lower rate of complications. They adjust the medications so that no weekend procedures are required. At these clinics the egg retrieval procedure is usually performed under a local anaesthetic instead of a general, so you would be awake. The advancements in low-cost IVF have dramatically improved over the last few years.

If you have time on your side of the biological clock and are able to save money specifically for fertility treatment, put that money aside. It will be such a relief knowing that you have this ready for treatment and that you won't have to be stressed about money when you are going through treatments.

Do a full review of all your personal expenses and see

what you can remove or cut down on. Call your bank to ask if you can get a cheaper interest rate on your home loan. It is recommended to do this every twelve to eighteen months as your bank will most likely never call you to say that interest rates have dropped. You have to get onto them and ask yourself. Another quick and easy saving is on insurance premiums; review your home and contents insurance amounts. Also, health insurance and life/income protection insurance— review these to make sure you know what your coverage and premiums are. A great organisation tool is Google Docs, just set up a basic spreadsheet and update as you go, and share this with your partner so that you both are involved.

Also, when you are in the zone of finances, this is a great time to research and get advice from a certified financial advisor. Let them know your starting point and that your goal is to start a family, but that you will require money for fertility treatments to do this. This is such a good time to review your financial situation and put a plan in place for the next five, ten, fifteen years. Yes, financial situations change, however it is so important to regularly review your finances and goals. It will give you direction and peace of mind.

If ongoing fertility treatment costs are getting out of hand, there is an Australian company called SuperCare where certain medical treatments, including IVF and surrogacy, can be paid for by your superannuation. You can apply for early release of super via Services Australia. It is highly recommended that you seek financial advice on this, but it is an option.

Get organised! If you do go through fertility treatment, there will be paperwork, receipts, refunds, medical tax thresholds, etc. Set up an email account just for fertility that you share with your partner and have your medical bills directed there. Or set up a subfolder within your everyday email account to store all of your fertility emails. Keep a basic Google Sheet of your treatment dates, cycle numbers, eggs retrieved and frozen embryos, etc. Keeping this basic information now will be a time saver in future; if you change doctors or clinics they need all your past medical information and you will have this in your Google documents.

It can be very tempting to add up ALL the money you have spent on fertility treatments, including the IVF, natural therapies, supplements, and fertility programs and think *What could I have bought with all this money?* But know that the money you have spent has been with good intent. It has been for the purpose of trying to bring a healthy baby into the world. And if that hasn't happened yet, know that the money already spent has been used for love, and that money is an energy that comes and goes, and that you can always get more money.

# staying sane tips

1. Look into the new low-cost IVF clinics as this format is expanding and their service offerings are increasing.

1. Review all your personal expenses, see what you can cut down and/or negotiate better premiums on.

2. Save up money specifically for IVF, because knowing you have your IVF savings will be a huge stress relief when going through treatments.

3. When planning for a baby it is a good time to seek financial advice from a certified professional. You have already gone through your expenses and with a professional you can review your goals and put a plan in place. This will give you direction.

4. If you cannot afford the ongoing medical expenses, SuperCare may be able to offer a portion of your superannuation to cover the costs of IVF or surrogacy.

5. Get organised for all the medical paperwork by setting up a special email address just for medical correspondence. Or set up a subfolder in your current email for all things medical. Keep a Google Sheet tracking all your cycle dates, numbers, treatments,

*medication, etc., as this will come in handy if you change doctors or clinics.*

6. *Know that what you have spent on all your fertility treatments and natural therapies has been for good purpose and out of pure love for your desire to bring a healthy baby into this world. If the thought of adding up all these costs comes to mind, know that because it is based on love, you can never put a dollar value on it. (Perhaps bring awareness to it but it is really priceless.)*

---

# 9
# Loony bin meds and operations

They say that laughter is the best medicine. However, when trying to have a baby, sometimes laughter is not enough and you have to take the medication as well. The medications come in many different shapes, sizes, brands and packaging and with different instructions. Some have to be taken with food, others one hour prior to food, some in the morning, during the day and some at night. Often there are instructions on the exact timing of a medication down to the minute it is to be administered.

The many different forms of these medications are nose sprays, tablets, injections, implants and pessaries. Also all the natural therapy meds, such as herbs that are boiled on the stove or in tablet form, supplements, drops under the tongue and those not to be taken with food or drinks.

With medications come side effects. Regularly there are headaches, mood swings, hot flushes, nausea, dizziness, abdominal discomfort, bloating, and bruises on the skin at the injection site. Wow, this sounds like fun, where do we sign up? Can't wait to get on that roller-coaster ride! And hopefully we don't end up at the divorce office from all this crazy excitement.

And when you are doing a full IVF cycle, after you have taken the daily stimulation injections to hopefully grow lots of good-quality eggs, then comes the egg pick-up day procedure, which usually involves fasting from a certain time the night before. And two nights prior to the pick-up day procedure is the big trigger injection, which is a special formula that will release the eggs. This is timed exactly to when your pick-up procedure is booked in for, down to the very minute. There cannot be any delays with this at all. So sync your calendars and put all alarms on, as you don't want to stuff up this very important schedule.

I had heard all the stories and read the trash magazine articles that IVF medications send you to the loony bin. That patients get emotional, have angry outbursts, are happy one minute and sad the next. That relationships get strained, and marriages bust up.

Therefore, on starting my very first IVF medication—which was the nose spray—I was bracing for the worst. Yes, I did get a few headaches to start with but no emotional outbursts. *Ok, tick that box,* I thought. I could safely move on to the next medication on the IVF cycle plan.

Next was the big one, the one I had feared for years. The one that I did hypnotherapy to get over. The daily egg stimulation injections.

The nurses had shown my husband how to administer the injections, what amount to use and where to put them in my body. The top of the thigh or stomach was advised. And the day came for the very first injection.

Now, my husband suffers from a hereditary shaky-hand condition where sometimes if he is a little stressed, his hands can shake a bit. Great! His hands were holding the big fat needle that was to be injected into me somehow. I was trying to stay calm and relaxed, taking big, deep breaths. I was in the lounge room watching *Twilight* to try and distract myself; hmm, maybe the vampire-sucking-blood movie wasn't the best choice! In he walks with the needle held upright in the air; I definitely didn't look directly at the needle but I could see it from the corner of my eye. Oh no, it looked quite a decent size. And in went the needle into my thigh. I took another deep breath, still trying my hardest to focus on Bella and Edward on the screen. I was bracing myself for the massive pain that I had been expecting. However, to my complete surprise and relief it didn't massively hurt; there was only a little sting, nowhere near as bad as I thought it would be. In my mind I had imagined that the needle would be in for, like, five minutes, but it was only about twenty seconds and then it was done.

OMG, what a huge relief. I had done it! I had survived the big needle injection into my thigh. I had this wave roll over me and the knots in my belly washed away. I felt so empowered after this, I now knew I could do this IVF cycle with all its needles and medications and we could finally have our baby.

Ok, now on to the second night, as we had to do the injections at the same time each night. This time, instead of injecting into the thigh, we tried the belly, as we thought that since the belly is softer and less muscley it should not sting. Again I took my position in the lounge room with the TV on as a distraction, and the injection went into my belly. Hmmm, that wasn't bad at all. I really only felt my husband squeezing my belly skin in his hands, didn't feel the actual needle and there was no stinging. What a huge relief. Finally I felt strong and in control, I could do this. My needle fear was gone—well, nearly. Each time the needle went in I had to really push my mind to focus on the TV and not on the fact that the needle was in my belly.

So this was our nightly routine for the next week and a half. So romantic! At least I got out of doing the dishes! I had to "rest and recover" in the lounge room after the injection, so Hubby cleaned up the kitchen after dinner whilst I was busy growing eggs.

With the injections I again was bracing for the side effects I had heard about in all the horror stories. However, I was very lucky and didn't suffer from any of these. I worked, I came home and rested, I went out walking and took it easy and thankfully I stayed sane. The worst would have been a few small bruises on my belly from where the injections went in, not every time though, just a few. At least it showed where the injections had gone in, so that the following night my husband could use a different patch of skin.

After about a week and a half of the regular injections came time for the big one ... the trigger injection. This needle has a lot more fluid. As mentioned, this has to be administered at a specific time down to the exact minute, so that the eggs can release just before the egg pick-up procedure approximately thirty-seven hours later. The type of needle was different and we didn't have any spare ones if it stuffed up. So there was a bit more pressure with this one. I had been feeling so confident with the other nightly injections that after a while I didn't need the TV on as a distraction. So this injection went into my belly and it stung, and the injection pen made a loud clicking sound so I couldn't ignore the fact that there was a big-arse needle in my belly. It felt like it took forever for it to go in ... *click, click, click*. The stinging continued all while the needle was in and then after it was finished the skin at the injection site was burning. It took about fifteen minutes for the burning sensation to fade away.

Wow, I had made it through the injection phase, I was so relieved. And I was so thankful I had my husband to administer the injections, as I know some friends who had to do that themselves because their husbands couldn't stand the sight of needles. I wouldn't know what to do if I had to read the needle instructions and inject it myself. Each night I would have had to drive to a chemist or a friend for them to jab me. I know one of my friends had to do the injections for another IVF friend, so I'm very grateful my hubby was able to do the injections and he did them really well, shaky hands and all.

Next was egg pick-up day. More needles. We arrived early in the morning at the IVF clinic, after I was not allowed to eat or drink anything. After sitting in the waiting area for a little while, we got split up. Oh no, this was the part where I am taken into the white, sterile hospital ward, while my husband stays in the familiar clinic where he has to produce his sperm sample. I got into my lovely hospital gown and lay on the bed and was wheeled into the waiting area just outside of the operating theatre. The anaesthetist came in to have a chat and get my veins ready. Oh, great, I have that small vein issue and hadn't been able to drink lots of water to pump them up. So they took a look at my veins and hmm'd and err'd under their breath … great. Finally they found the spot at the back of my hand and got the stuff set up and left me alone again.

By this stage I was getting really scared and feeling all alone, with only strangers around me wanting to put needles in me. The anticipation of the anaesthetist coming back in and putting the needle into my hand was starting to freak me out. I was trying to have a baby but I was also feeling like a baby, crying over getting a needle!

By the time the anaesthetist walked back in I had tears rolling down my face. The normal pre-op process is that the anaesthetist has the vein ready with the needle in place, waiting to administer the sleepy-time meds. And you get wheeled into the theatre and are transferred to the operating table. Normally you are still awake and can help lift yourself from the comfy bed and onto the table, and then the anaesthetist will start the meds and you go fast asleep and the operation begins. However, as I was so upset the anaesthetist gave me something straight away to send me into la-la land before I got wheeled into the operating theatre. Thank goodness, as la-la land was so much better!

When I woke up, I didn't know where I was for a moment as the drugs were still wearing off. However, when I came around, I felt relief. Such pure relief that I had made it. The doctors had done their thing and I really didn't want to know what they had been doing or where—just that I had made it to the other side. I also kind of felt proud of myself that I had made it through the physically hardest parts of the IVF cycle, the daily injections, hormonal meds and egg retrieval operation. These were all the hardest parts … so I thought.

I ended up staying in the recovery room for ages as I get low blood pressure. At first I was starving, so I ate some cheese and crackers. Next I felt so good I got out of bed and dressed, however that wave feeling started where I felt so light-headed that I nearly passed out, so had to lie down again. This happened numerous times, I would feel good, get up and then sit down again. However, finally the blood pressure was better. My husband was beside me and we walked out to the car.

I am a very easy vomiter. If there were a medal for vomiting, I reckon I could be in the running. I can have a slight headache, walk to the bathroom, do a quick vomit and walk back out like "nothing special going on here". On the long drive home I felt relief that we were nearly back to our house, but two minutes from home, very suddenly I wasn't feeling good. This time it wasn't the low blood pressure but the nausea instead. I got my husband to stop the car and on the side of the road I threw up in the gutter like there was no tomorrow. Yes, it was a good look; I was hanging out the car, throwing up in the gutter. Better in the gutter than in our car.

After that I felt so much better. Instant relief. It had been a combination of everything I had been through over the last few weeks getting out of my body: the anxiety, emotional roller-coaster, stress, hormone-stimulating medications, fear and anticipation.

When we got home, we got comfy on the couch. It was like our own little haven after the sterile hospital environment. We watched movies and I talked with my mum and sisters to let them know how things went.

Over the next couple of days I felt fine, there was no pain, but my belly was very bloated. I had to wear light clothes and definitely nothing with a tight waistband, and drank heaps of fluids.

After the second day at home I felt really good, so I went back to work, but made sure I wore a very loose skirt due to my bloated belly. I really loved my job and always had heaps of laughs in the office so I happily went in.

All the while our eggs and sperm had fertilised and our embryos were now growing. It was a strange feeling to think that finally my egg and my husband's sperm had met and were growing together, as I had never had this before. It felt nice to know our future babies had just been conceived, even though it was via a laboratory Petri dish … we didn't care how.

By the time of my last full IVF cycle, I felt like a veteran at mixing normal life with fertility treatment—one minute getting my eggs retrieved and the next having a birthday party for my husband. I'd done it all before and knew that I didn't need to stop living just because I was going through an IVF cycle. I just carried on like whatever.

However, this particular IVF cycle I had the egg pick up the day before my husband's thirty-eighth birthday. And the day after I went back to work, but by lunch time I wasn't feeling that crash hot, so I drove myself the thirty minutes home. It was a Friday and on the drive home the bloated pain I had been experiencing got really bad. It was all hard when you pressed around my rib cage and each breath I took was so painful that I started crying whilst driving home. Driving whilst in heaps of pain and crying is really not recommended, I definitely was not a safe driver that day.

So that Friday night I took myself to bed very early. However, at midnight I woke up and was in so much pain just trying to breathe. Each breath in caused a sharp pain as my belly was all swollen due to the many eggs they had retrieved. My husband called the hospital as that was in the post-operation instructions, and they suggested I come in. Well that was another forty-five-minute drive and when you are feeling pain from any sudden movement, you feel every single little bump in the road like you have never felt them before. I would brace for each corner and stoplight.

Once we got to the hospital, I had to run them through what procedure I had and how many eggs they had retrieved. Everything checked out ok and they gave me some medication for the pain. We stayed in the hospital for a few hours and I was released to go home with pain meds and told to get some rest.

The next day I felt ok in the early morning, but after taking the codeine I felt sick and threw up. However, by the early afternoon I felt great again.

As it was my husband's birthday weekend, we had organised with a few close friends to go to the movies. These friends knew

I was going through an IVF cycle and that it was a bit touch and go if I would make it to the movies. However, I got ready. I was in pain, but I didn't want to admit that. I did my hair and makeup beautifully (have I mentioned that I am a qualified makeup artist?) and took some codeine and off we drove to the movies. We met our friends there and went inside. It was a space movie and I actually hate space movies, but again it was my husband's birthday and I was trying to enjoy it for him.

On the drive in I had felt nauseous, and after being in the movie theatre for a little while I went out to the bathrooms. When I got into the corridor, I knew I wasn't going to make it as the bathrooms were a bit of a distance. I had previously laughed at my ability to throw up easily. However, on this occasion, when I was walking super fast down the corridor, past all the life-size cardboard cut-outs of Hollywood stars ... I did a little chuck up and tried to catch it in my hand (not sure what my hand was going to do). Yes, me in my beautiful dress, with nice makeup and long hair styled with big loose curls, trying to catch my vomit in my hand. And guess what? I didn't get any in my hair or on my face. I'm so impressed with my skill. Not sure if I can put that on my résumé though!

Thankfully there had been no one walking down the corridor at that exact time and I hightailed it to the bathrooms, where again I did a beautiful ladylike vomit. And once I got all that out, I felt so much better. I washed and left the bathrooms, and saw my husband waiting outside for me. He was concerned, but I told him that after the numerous throw ups I felt fine. We walked back up the corridor and again, thankfully, there was no one walking around at that time—I really did time that well. However, there were two young movie attendants chatting at the cleaning cupboard. On the walk back I saw my puke on the carpet on the other side of the corridor … as you do. And I reluctantly told Hubby that it belonged to me. So my husband told the movie attendants that it looked like someone had thrown up just down the corridor, hinting that the "someone" had to be someone else, and definitely not me. They thanked him hesitantly and got their buckets and off they walked to clean it up. In that moment I felt so bad for them that they had to clean up my vomit.

So in we walked back to our seats and continued watching the space movie. I had no idea what was going on but Matthew McConaughey was in it. And about another twenty minutes later I wasn't feeling good, so we left. I felt so bad as we had to leave the others there and one of our friends was with us so he had to leave the movie early as well. And after that ordeal I never took codeine again as I finally realised that it was making me sick!

So when you start on the medical intervention journey, the most important thing is to be kind to yourself and treat yourself and your partner as the priority. You are on this journey together; if it works you will be parents together, and if it does not you will be able to go on other great adventures together.

As the amazing Melissa Ambrosini says in her book *Open Wide*, we need to express *crystal clear communication*. This is so important and especially so when you are going through IVF, as there are many more outside elements happening. Whatever you are feeling, communicate this to your partner. Even if sometimes you might not know how to express what you are feeling in words, just connect with them via a hug.

In our busy lifestyles where it always seems to be go, go, go, doing an IVF cycle or a natural fertility program will make you more aware of this unnecessary busyness. It will make you more conscious of slowing down and being kind to yourself, which is a great thing. There were multiple times I had gone back to work the very next day after an egg pick-up procedure. On my second IVF cycle I had gone back to work the next day and we all went out to lunch as it was the birthday of one of my work friends and I remember sitting very uncomfortably on the extremely hard wooden chair eating Thai food, but I didn't enjoy the yummy food as I was in pain because my belly was swollen and it was hard to breathe. There would be no way I would push myself like that now as I have learnt the hard way that we need to take time for ourselves, for healing and rejuvenation.

When it comes to work, the best thing is to let your manager know. And they will surprise you with their understanding. My first boss was very understanding and would ask me questions about how I was going. And my second boss, well he and his wife had been through IVF to have their baby themselves, so he knew from a male point of view the challenges. They were both so supportive. Otherwise I would have had to sneak around and not be completely truthful to go to the medical appointments. And they would probably have thought that I was looking for another job or something.

When you are on the daily injections, let your partner take care of the cooking and cleaning. If the needles freak you out, distract yourself by watching something good on Netflix. Laze on the lounge and make sure your belly is all soft for when the needle goes in. And absolutely don't look at the needle! Put a warm heat bag on your belly beforehand also really helps with reducing the sting and it had a nice comforting feeling.

On egg pick-up day, if your nervous or dreading it, tell your doctor and nurses that you don't like the operating theatre and ask them to give you something to make you doze off before they wheel you in. This will make the whole experience a lot better. And after the egg pick-up, drink, drink, drink. No, definitely not coffee or wine! Get stuck into water for hydration and electrolyte powders mixed in water and sip these all day. Also, you may not feel like it, but keep moving in the days after egg pick up. When I made the mistake of going straight back to work and sitting at my desk, this was actually the worst thing I could have done as you need to keep moving to decrease the swollen belly and help with breathing. Gentle movement is good, like walking, light stretches, and getting into a warm pool or ocean. Draw a warm bath at home with essential oils and read a good book. Make sure you get outside into nature and let the sun soak into your skin whilst taking nice, big, deep belly breaths. This time is for you to rejuvenate and heal. So soak up the goodness as these might just be the very last days before you fall pregnant.

# staying sane tips

1. *Be kind to yourself and your partner. Share this journey with crystal-clear communication. Don't assume your partner knows what you are thinking, let them in.*

2. *Slow down, smell the roses and be gentle on your body. Especially when you are on daily injections. Take time out for yourself, rest and rejuvenate. You are human and humans need rest.*

3. *Let your manager at work know. You cannot control everything, such as the timing of those early morning appointments. And you might be happily surprised by your manager's support and understanding.*

4. *On egg pick-up day, ask the anaesthetist to give you something before being wheeled into the theatre as this will calm you down and make the hospital experience more positive.*

5. *Rest and drink plenty of water and electrolytes after the egg pick up. Move your body in gentle movements through light stretching and walking.*

# 10

# Watching paint dry and ground zero

Waiting! Really the whole experience of trying to get pregnant is about waiting. We wait for a new monthly cycle to start, wait for ovulation to do some serious baby making, wait for that positive pregnancy test, wait for the excitement of telling family and friends at the safe twelve-week mark, wait to be able to buy baby clothes and nursery furniture. And when that doesn't go to plan, we wait for doctor appointments, wait for cycle days to start, wait for timed injections, wait for egg pick-up days, wait for the eggs to fertilise, wait for day-five blastocyst embryos to grow, wait for embryo transfer days, and then there's the biggest wait of all—the two-week wait, or the waiting game. Not sure why it was ever referred to as a game. I guess maybe because there are winners and losers.

And after all that waiting, if you are lucky to have a positive pregnancy test, you wait for the eight-week scan, followed by the twelve-week scan and then graduate to the big people's obstetrician. However, if that pregnancy test turns up a big, fat negative and you feel like you are back at ground zero, it is still a waiting game. Waiting for your body to heal, waiting for your heart to recover, waiting to get that inner spark back.

Ground zero can be the biggest kick in the guts ever. You have put in everything to try to have a baby. Your health, your body, your time, your money, your positive energy, your relationships, your work, your social life. Basically your life is on hold, in limbo, in an IVF bubble, spinning around hamster-wheel-style, chasing something that is right in front of you but you just can't get that bite. Real life gets put on hold. You are flattened at ground zero. Will you ever see the light again, ever truly smile and laugh again? Ever enjoy Mother's or Father's Day again?

During my life I have had my share of challenges that have flattened me, but I have always had a glass-half-full attitude. I just get back up, dust myself off and get on with it. I deal with it at the time, learn from it and move on. There is just so much in life to experience. And this is how I dealt with the two-week waits and negative pregnancy tests.

Five days after my first egg retrieval procedure, it was time for the embryo transfer. *This could be my pregnancy day,* I thought. It was kind of exciting to think that this could be the day I finally fell pregnant, even if it wasn't the most romantic of settings. So we headed back into the clinic and had a chat with the embryologist, who talked about the embryos and how they develop. From the embryos they pick the best one—the one they can tell is technically the best from looking under a microscope. They even printed us out a photo of the embryo. It is a strange feeling looking at a picture of your own embryo, as it could really be your baby's first photo.

Off we walked into the embryo transfer room where they ask your name and date of birth a number of times. I happily answered them as many times as they asked, I wanted them to be sure they were transferring the correct embryo. The embryo transfer room is probably not the most romantic place in the world, as there is the IVF doctor, the embryologist and a nurse or two. However, before you know it, the embryo is in place.

You would think that after years of trying to fall pregnant, going through all the natural fertility programs under the sun and numerous IUI cycles, and finally doing IVF, that you would feel it. You know, you would feel the embryo snuggling into your uterus wall and starting to grow into a baby. Well no, you don't feel anything. I was scared to get up off the bed in case it fell out! Then you change and walk right back out, get in the car and go home. It all happens so quickly; after all the planning and waiting, the actual embryo transfer procedure is the quickest.

When I was getting in and out of the car, I was trying not to use any of my stomach muscles as I was trying to keep the little embryo in place. And when I started to laugh I was like, oh no, I don't want to laugh it out! And don't even think about sneezing … OMG, all these little things I was thinking. I became very aware of my stomach. I didn't want to strain, bend or move in a strange way. However, all this is crap, just my mind going into overdrive.

## THE TWO-WEEK WAIT

The IVF clinic tips after the embryo transfer were very limited; it was just *Go home and in two weeks' time, get a blood test.* How are you supposed to just relax? However, my Chinese medicine natural therapist provided so many helpful tips: eat and drink warm foods, do not lift anything heavy, do not stretch up (therefore no hanging the clothes on the clothesline), have a warm bath or shower but not too hot, no vigorous exercise, watch funny movies and laugh.

So then begins the waiting … the two-week wait. This part really does sound easy. Just chill out and relax and you'll fall pregnant. But it's not so easy, as it is the only thing that you think about all day every day. Even when I really tried hard to think of other things, it just kept creeping back in. I would laze around for a few days, watched movies and read.

On this first embryo transfer I ended up missing my nephew's christening, which was a four-hour drive away. So that was also challenging as I really wanted to be out and about with my family, but again had to rest.

After the long weekend of resting and watching movies at home, we drove down the coast as we had booked an apartment near the beach. I lazed around the pool and read books. However, on the eighth day post embryo transfer, I started bleeding. This was a complete shock. I was supposed to get a blood test at two weeks exactly after the embryo transfer, I even had the script for that waiting. So why was I bleeding now? I didn't understand and definitely wasn't advised about this beforehand. I called the clinic and the nurse advised that this sometimes happens and it might even be implantation bleeding. So keep resting, she said, and get your blood test done on day fourteen.

So back home we drove and I had my blood test. The nurse called that afternoon to tell me what I already knew, that it was negative, I wasn't pregnant. My possible implantation bleeding had become a full-on period. I knew I wasn't pregnant, but the nurse ringing was just another kick in the guts.

From this first IVF cycle we also didn't get any frozen embryos. So this negative really felt like ground zero. I remember lying on my bed in the dark in the fetal position and crying my heart out, I just couldn't stop crying. I had been so cool and calm during this process, I remember feeling great that the IVF drugs didn't make me loopy, I did the needle thing well, and I went back to work after the egg pick-up procedure. On this negative-result day I was floored; I had gone through so much preparation, done all the appointments and early mornings, rested when I was supposed to, and didn't drink alcohol or coffee, but it still didn't work. This was supposed to be our baby time, a celebration, but it was only sadness.

So I threw myself back into work, which was good as it was the busiest time of the year, and I went out and played softball every second Saturday. And four months later I was ready to get back out there and start another IVF cycle. This time our doctor changed the brand of the injection medication and on egg pick-up day they retrieved double the amount of eggs than my first time. However, it isn't about the number but the quality. We had two embryos transferred this time and had three embryos to freeze. Wow, this felt amazing, I was so much more confident and relaxed on this cycle.

However, maybe I did push myself a little bit to be the perfect IVF patient whilst still being the perfect corporate worker. I had had twenty eggs retrieved but still went back to work the next day. Yes, my belly was bloated and I was drinking water with electrolytes like crazy. However, my work was so busy and I didn't want to disappoint anyone, always the people pleaser.

One morning I woke up and had these very strong abdominal pains. I had never had these before and never felt them again. The next day, which was only day seven post the two embryos being transferred, I started bleeding. I still waited for the blood test on day fourteen, which again was negative. However, I didn't get upset this time, I think I was just focused on the next transfer as I knew I had embryos in the freezer. It was like I had my game face on, just focusing on the end goal and doing anything to get there.

I still wonder to this day if those sharp abdominal pains were the embryos removing themselves from my uterus wall. Maybe I was pregnant, maybe they actually did implant into my uterus this time. But did I work too hard, push myself to do everything? If I had rested more after the transfer, would I be a mum and have a child in school today? I will always wonder but I'll never know for sure.

During this time, the hand-me-down baby clothes, blankets, bottles, and a beautiful timber cradle that had all the white lace trimmings on it all got taken to the op shop. I had held on to it all for years; even when we moved house, it moved with us. But I just could not look at it anymore. I felt sad, like a failure. I had all this beautiful baby stuff ready and waiting but no baby.

Also during this year of IVF, I went to a spiritual and psychic fair with some friends. It was supposed to be a fun day out learning about new meditations, reiki and crystal healing, etc. However, I did a psychic reading for the first time ever and the psychic told me that he didn't see me having a baby for a while. I was really annoyed at this because I was just about to start a new round of IVF. What could that mean? My friends were reassuring me that psychic readings often get the timing wrong. I wanted a baby so badly and this reading really got to me. *Do I stop my next round of IVF I have booked in because of a psychic reading?* I started questioning myself and our baby plans. In the end I let the psychic reading go and got stuck into our next IVF cycle.

When you start IVF, there is this feeling and expectation that this works, and that it works every time. How many times had I read in the trash magazines that celebrities and people fell pregnant on IVF? I just thought it worked. One celebrity that I followed had fallen pregnant on her third cycle and when I got to number three I thought *Yep, this is the one, because IVF works and it absolutely works by the third go.*

So on to our third cycle we went. This was *the one*, I could just feel it. And even better, this cycle we had embryos in the freezer. Woohoo, this felt so good. Kinda like a backup boyfriend, just hovering in the corner and waiting for my instructions to jump. No more daily injections, no egg pick-up operations or bloated, painful belly for three days afterwards. We just cut the queue and went straight to the embryo transfer day. And again I had two transferred.

I tried to rest and relax for a few days afterwards, but I did go back to work and tried to take it easy. And yet again I started bleeding before the day-fourteen blood test, which I still did and yes, the result was negative.

I was kind of getting used to this feeling of being knocked down. The worst day during the two-week wait was when I would start bleeding early and have to tell my husband that I didn't think it worked. I knew he felt helpless. He said to me lovingly many times that he wished he was the one getting the injections and operations, as he knew I struggled with them.

Another thing that can be challenging during the two-week wait is pretending. One Christmas we were having an early family lunch at my in-laws' place the weekend before Christmas Day. I had just had an embryo transfer so couldn't drink alcohol. Before going to the lunch I looked up mocktail recipes online and liked the look of the Virgin Mary drink.

I hadn't really told many people that I was doing an IVF cycle as I much preferred the idea of just having a *Surprise, I'm pregnant!* moment like most other couples get to do.

At the Christmas lunch I was drinking the Virgin Marys, which weren't that great, and was trying to enjoy myself, but I kept thinking about the embryo transfer and wondering if it had taken. The table discussion turned a little and back then I didn't really speak up that much around the in-laws, but on this particular occasion I did and was disagreeing with the others.

And then I got up from the table and walked off midway through the meal. I would never usually do that as I used to be the quiet one, but off I stormed. Really I was just struggling with pretending to live a normal life while going through all these crazy emotions.

The anticipation of the embryo transfer and the two-week wait can easily get to you, and I just had everything bottled up. When I was at work I was all cool and calm, but at that family lunch I just couldn't keep the mixed emotions in anymore they had to get out, and I did feel a lot better afterwards. Also, most of the family ended up knowing that I was on a cycle anyway and they didn't care that I had stormed off, they just wanted to know that I was ok.

Straight after the third negative, we were ready to go ahead with a fresh IVF cycle as we just knew it was going to work. It was December and we wanted to start the new year pregnant. So off we went merrily for a full IVF cycle, more needles, operations, belly bloating. This round my doctor didn't want to stimulate me as much, rather focus on the quality of the eggs. Again I had two embryos transferred, but this time only made it to five days before I started bleeding.

What the heck was going on? With each transfer cycle I seemed to start bleeding earlier. This one I remember very well as it was Christmas. We had planned to have Christmas with the family at the beach, and I had never done a beach Christmas before. So we packed all the food, presents, decorations, music, bonbons, and also togs, towels, the surf ski, etc. It was just the two of us at home on Christmas morning when I woke up and

Santa had brought me a big, fat negative. All I wanted was a baby and I got my period instead on Christmas morning. Merry fucking Christmas! But I got up and put on a pretty dress, we packed the car and my husband drove us to the beach. In the car I was receiving all these lovely Happy Christmas messages from family and friends, but all I wanted to write back was Merry Fucking Christmas.

And that rounded out our first year of IVF. Four cycles with seven embryos transferred and a big, fat nothing to show for it. Oh, but we did have two frozen embryos from different cycles, therefore we felt one ounce of relief in that. However, the beach Christmas negative cycle really hurt. I had put on a brave face, but I was crushed inside. I would wear the brave face mask so well. But it wasn't just Christmas Day, it was Boxing Day and basically the whole week between Christmas and New Year. Normally I love this time of year as you are around family and friends whilst eating everything. But this one just felt off, like there was a dark shadow hovering over me that I couldn't shake.

Even though I knew I had those two frozen embryos, all the following year I just could not go there. I needed a break, a new focus, and something other than a baby to look forward to. And that became our year off, with my husband getting a new job and us planning our big white Christmas holiday overseas with our friends. With planning this holiday I just really wanted Christmas to be better than it had been the previous year. I wanted to remove the Merry Fucking Christmas memories in my head and replace them with Merry Wonderful White Christmas.

As previously explained, after we had a few years off I found Investigative Doctor and went on to do five months of back-to-back Zoladex 3.6 mg implant injections. This was to reduce the adenomyosis in my uterus wall, which should help an embryo to implant. Thankfully I did this during winter as it basically sends you into a pre-menopausal state. And we all know what that means ... hot flushes. These are really strange; I would be sitting at my desk in air conditioning with a jacket on and suddenly feel this wave of heat go through me. And off came the jacket. But I wasn't doing anything like physical exercise, just typing. It did stop my period, which was weird. The implants just went into my belly and for me, who's not a fan of needles, this was actually not painful at all. I don't mind needles going in, I just don't really like blood tests where they put a needle into your vein—still not a fan of that, like, ever!

From the five months of implants, I went straight into a frozen embryo transfer. Just one embryo this time. But I started bleeding five days later.

By this stage a negative result was kind of expected, like if I actually did fall pregnant it would be a complete and utter surprise.

I still had one embryo in the freezer and after doing all the Zoladex implants, I wanted to get this transfer done asap. However, as mentioned in Chapter 4, my awesome investigative doctor retired, so on to a new doctor we went and we did this embryo transfer on a natural cycle, which is where you have your normal monthly cycle and on your ovulation day the thawed embryo is transferred. And yes, I started bleeding ten days later. Oh well, that was all my frozen embryos used up with still no baby. Back to ground zero again, and I was getting older and more frustrated by the whole baby thing.

So this is when we went onto the VIP fertility program with the naturopath in Ireland for the next five months. We did a full IVF cycle that produced our very best-ever eggs and fertilisations, and the most blastocyst embryos ever. And we had one super good-looking embryo transferred, but on day ten I started bleeding … again. I did feel gutted, and back at ground zero again, but I felt comfort in knowing I had five good-looking embryos in the freezer. There was also a part of me that knew I would never do a full fresh IVF cycle again. It was just this inner feeling that I couldn't go through all the needles and egg retrievals again.

So as a wrap up, we had four full IVF cycles and three frozen cycles, with ten embryos transferred. We could have had ten kids by now. And we still have five embryos in the freezer.

Sometimes I think, if a particular cycle had been successful, we would have children in school by now. We would have liked to have had two kids. I wonder what school they would have gone to, and what their interests would have been.

We have had my hopes go up, down and sideways many times. But eventually we started digging our way back out, moving one rock at a time, seeing that sunlight after the rain, taking that big breath of fresh air and relishing the feeling of life again.

The two-week wait is where your mind can go into overdrive and play tricks on you. All the questions run through your brain.

Are you pregnant or are you not? Is that twinge a pregnancy twinge or a premenstrual twinge? Are my boobs sore due to pregnancy or PMS? Is that nausea feeling pregnancy? Is that weird food craving pregnancy?

This is where your mental strength will be tested. Allow your mind to think of the above things, but for only one time per day. And when that thought creeps back in for the second, fourth, sixth, twentieth time, tell that thought that you have already had it today and that you are not going to have it again. This will get easier; you need to mentally tell yourself to change your thinking. Or do the rubber-band trick and snap the band when the thought creeps back again.

### Three things you can do instead of watch paint dry

*1. Projects*

Get stuck into projects. When trying to survive the two-week wait, yes, do all the usual rest and relaxation things like watching movies and reading good books, but what are the things that you have always really wanted to do? It might be doing that online course on photography or essential oils, organising your kitchen pantry, learning about Indian cooking spices, listening to an audiobook on decluttering, or finally getting around to doing that online photo book from your last holiday. Or you might start a new passion project as a side hustle, such as crafting and selling items on Etsy. Use this time to do the things, learnings and projects that you have often thought of but never got around to doing. This will help distract you, as Netflix can only do so much.

## 2. Gratitude and journaling

When we get stuck in our heads, we often think of all the things that could go wrong or all the negative things in the world. If you reverse this and start to be grateful for all the good things in your life, you will start to see a change in your perspective. Every morning or night write down in your journal three things you are grateful for. At the start of this process, it might be the usual things, but dig deeper and you will notice more things to be grateful for. With time this will help you see the positive in more situations.

## 3. Connect

If you are at home during your two-week wait and your partner is at work, it might be easy to withdraw from your friends. However, now is the time to call your friends, as even just a five-minute convo will make you feel better. If you know your friends are busy, send them a message and say that you are at home and ask if they give you a call when they have a few spare minutes. And if you have any friends who have gone through IVF, call them and let them know you are in the two-week wait. They might have some tips you have not thought of. Just reaching out and connecting is such a powerful thing.

## GROUND ZERO

Ground zero is a strange place, as you have just put in so much energy, time and money with nothing to show for it, apart from medical bills. If you are lucky, you might have some frozen embryos as a consolation prize.

Failure with IVF can be a very lonely thing. If you play sport and you lose a game, you have your teammates or coach to share in the failure, and the usual deconstruction of the game and what you can do differently next time. With a failed IVF, let it out, feel your emotions with your partner, talk about it with your close family and friends. Get it all out, write it down in your journal. What you are feeling, thinking or struggling with. See this as a form of release, to get out all the stuff in your head and in your heart. Release and let it go.

Be gentle with yourself and when the time comes—and you will know when it is time—deconstruct the game with your doctor and fertility coach. Go over what you think worked and what you think didn't work. Let them know all your symptoms and reactions to the medications, herbs, etc. If the doctor just wants to go again and you want more investigation, tell them, or research another doctor who specialises in your exact area. The patient/doctor relationship is so important, so make sure you feel good about your next game plan.

If you are going through IVF around Christmas time, make sure you surround yourself with family and friends. Invite everyone to go to the beach or park. Get inspired to cook Christmas food or craft decorations. Get yourself into the Christmas spirit rather than withdrawing alone, as you will feel so much better.

To help with that positive spirit or spark, get stuck into reading positive books and blogs or listening to podcasts. It is amazing what listening to an awesome ten-minute podcast whilst driving to the shops or walking can do for your mental state and energy.

We are only human. Sometimes in life, things go to plan and things are awesome, but other times things go to shit and we find ourselves heartbroken at ground zero.

However, even at ground zero, this thing too shall pass. You will start to see the sun, start to see the beauty, start to feel that smile, start to feel like laughing, and yes, start to feel like dancing again.

# staying sane tips

1.  Strengthen your mind during the two-week embryo wait. When the Am I/am I not pregnant *thoughts come in*, only let your mind think of those thoughts once a day. And when they pop up again, tell yourself that you have already had that thought today, and let it pass.

2.  Start learning those things you have been putting off. Invest time in all the projects that you have wanted to do. This will help strengthen your mind and may even open new opportunities.

3.  Write down in your journal three different things you are grateful for each day. This will help shift your mindset to automatically see the positive and beauty in each day.

4.  Connect with your close friends and family. Reach out and send messages and make calls. Share with your besties how you are really going.

5.  If your two-week results are negative, let yourself feel it. As hard as this can be, feel it, let the emotions out and with time they will pass. Share this with your partner, as they will be feeling it too.

6. *Deconstruct the game plan with your doctor and natural therapist. Ask questions, tell the doctor all your symptoms and work out a game plan for your next go.*

7. *If it is the holiday season, surround yourself with family and friends. Plan outings, get inspired by cooking and decorating in holiday themes. This will light that spark inside you.*

8. *Do things that spark positive energy inside you. Read inspiring books and blogs and listen to amazing podcasts that light you up. This will shift your perspective and help you see the light.*

# 11

# Comparisonitis

*Stay in your own lane. Comparison kills creativity and joy.*
— Brené Brown

What's with all the "my family" stick figure stickers on all the cars! When I drive anywhere I see them and then I start to compare myself to the stranger in the car in front of me. I count up how many stickers they have. Is it Mum, Dad and one kid, three kids or five kids? Is there a dog, is there a cat. I seem to really look at them and compare myself. If it's just one person with a dog, I'm like *Yeah, I have one up on them* as I have a dog *and* a husband. But if it's a couple with two or three kids, I'm like, *Ok* … a feeling of lacking creeps in as I don't have as much as they do.

When we were young, we would play with Barbie dolls, Cabbage Patch Kids and Barbie houses. The dolls would all look the same; they'd have the same faces and bodies with the only difference being their hair or outfit. We would play with our Barbie dolls with our friends and swap clothes, but by comparison the dolls were all the same.

When we hit puberty, we would compare ourselves to our friends; who was wearing a bra and who was not. It was like a race to get older and to look older. Funny how now as adults it is all about who looks younger!

And then we compare our weddings, from the groom to the engagement ring, the wedding dress, venue, guests, food, music, speeches, and even the honeymoon destination. So naturally we compare when we get to the next big step of pregnancy and babies. Who out of our friends is pregnant, who is glowing and who is struggling with pregnancy?

If falling pregnant becomes a challenge, it can be easy to start comparing yourself to family, friends, colleagues, your social media feed, celebrities in trash mags and even other patients waiting in the doctor's office. You can even compare yourself in online fertility and pregnancy chat rooms where many avatars will request your age, your partner's age, how long you have been trying to fall pregnant, how many IUI and IVF cycles you have done, how many frozen embryos you have—and it goes on and on, all just about numbers and more numbers. There is no heart or soul in these avatar signatures.

We moved when I was thirteen years old from a country town where there were 120 kids in my high school to a new area where there were seven hundred kids in my new school. All the cool kids were wearing Doc Martens and up until then I hadn't even known what a Doc Marten was. But suddenly I wanted them just because everyone else had them. And I thought to fit in I needed them.

Comparing myself to others is something I have always

seemed to do. I have even compared myself to my own mother; when my mum was thirty years old, she had had five children. So by the time I was around thirty, I thought I really should have had one or two kids by now.

Also, each year I would compare my current self to the self I wanted to be the following year. Each birthday I would think to myself that by my next birthday I would be pregnant, or be a mum. That I would be celebrating the next Mother's Day as a mum. And at that next Christmas we would have presents under our tree from Santa for our baby. I would compare all these milestones I was currently living with that future milestone in the following year. Always comparing and never really living in the moment.

I compared myself to celebrities, which is so silly to think of now, as they don't really live in the real everyday world that most of us do. If it was a celebrity who had done IVF, and it had taken them three cycles to fall pregnant, I would think that my third cycle would be a success. If I read in the trash mags that a celebrity had fallen pregnant on their first cycle of IVF, I would compare myself to them and think that they were not worthy of infertility warrior status. In the article they would describe how difficult doing IVF was but that on their first cycle they fell pregnant and they now have a beautiful bouncing baby, and there would be all these happy pictures displayed in the magazine. But I would think to myself that they were not worthy, that you have to do lots of IVF cycles and go through all the ups and downs to wear that warrior badge of honour. This is so harsh when I think about it now, as anyone who goes through IVF is a warrior and can wear that badge with honour.

One day I was sitting in the lunch room at work, flicking through a magazine, and who do I see? None other than my very first IVF doctor, the kind doctor in a two-page article. She was holding a baby so I madly start reading and discovered that she had gone through IVF to have this baby. She had previously had four kids, but in her new marriage they wanted a baby together so she ended up having IVF at forty-one years old and now had a new baby. The article stated that now she really understood all the physical and emotional challenges that her IVF patients have gone through as she had experienced it herself.

However, at the time that I read this article I was very much in the world of comparisonitis and I thought that there was no way she really understood; she had previously had four children and was already a mother, so how could she possibly understand other patients who were trying to have a baby? How could she compare herself to an IVF fertility warrior who is trying to fall pregnant for the first time and hopefully become a mum, when she was already a mum? I couldn't see past this.

However, now I think it is great that she spoke up about her IVF experience and I understand that each IVF patient has their own journey and story to tell, regardless of whether they are a mother or not.

I did struggle with sympathising with other IVF patients who already had a child and were trying for their second. I had full-on comparisonitis, always comparing my IVF journey to others'.

My friend and I went to a Christmas in July dinner with our IVF meet-up group at this beautiful restaurant. The dinner had been organised and the meals were already paid for by the IVF organisers. There were four of us girls in the car together and we were all madly chatting and laughing on the ride to the restaurant. When we walked inside, the restaurant looked so cosy and we started chatting to some other IVF people. We would chat about where we were on our journey, who our doctor was, what cycle we were on. I was more drawn to the people who had not had any children yet, as that was me, so we had common ground. If I spoke with someone who had already had a baby through IVF and was trying for their second, I would kind of move myself away as I was completely in that comparison world.

It would have been beneficial to chat with the people who were trying for their second as they were real-life examples of how IVF can be a success. But I was in that closed-off mindset of comparison and I couldn't see this.

When we all sat down to dinner, directly across from us was a pregnant woman. *Oh great*, I thought. I go to an IVF group dinner to discuss my challenges with trying to fall pregnant and I'm reminded of my lack of a baby by a pregnant woman sitting directly opposite me. Oh, and then she started to talk. And talk she did. We discovered that she was pregnant with not her first or second child, but her fifth! What the! Did she have the right restaurant? This was an IVF group dinner, not a parents group dinner. She talked the entire meal and explained that she and her husband had three children when they were first married.

However, when the children were leaving home after high school, she got empty-nest syndrome and they did IVF to have their fourth child. And after having him they had spare frozen embryos and they could not bring themselves to destroy them, so she was now pregnant with their fifth child. And she laughed that she still had more frozen embryos and would probably try for yet another.

My girlfriends and I were sitting across from her in disbelief. And in the car ride home we had a bit of a laugh about this. Not once did this woman ask us about our IVF journeys, it was all about her and her five kids and frozen embryos. Maybe she was just after the free meal. Were we comparing ourselves to her? Absolutely! Underneath our laugher and disbelief, did we want to be the ones pregnant at an IVF group dinner? Hell yeah. That comparisonitis can really bring out the worst in us at times.

Another support vehicle is the IVF online chat room. These are so handy as you can chat wherever and whenever. So if I was in need of some support from people who were going through the same things as I was and at the same time, I found logging in online sometimes helpful. However, I never really felt any better when I logged off and the main reason for this was again that comparisonitis.

I would compare myself to every one of the avatars. If they were older than me, I would feel good as I was younger and had more good-quality eggs and more fertile years. If I was older, I would feel bad as I would have poorer-quality eggs and fewer years to have a baby. If they had done fewer IVF cycles but had had a baby, I would feel jealous, but if they had done more cycles with no baby, I would feel ok.

I think the reason I felt these things was that I was only interacting with them online, so there was no depth or personal connection for me. It seemed like everyone was just striving to have a baby, asking which clinic or doctor had the best reviews, but there was no soul or raw emotion.

What's with all the talk of numbers on the baby making train?

When we first went to the IVF clinic, they asked all the usual questions, our ages, dates of birth, blood types and the results of sperm counts. How many years we had been trying to fall pregnant, etc. And when you are going through an IVF cycle, there are all the ultrasounds where they record how many egg follicles are growing in the ovaries.

Then on the egg retrieval day, when I would wake up from the operation in the recovery room, I would look at the back of my wrist and there would be a big number written in black marker pen—the number of eggs they had retrieved.

The next day the clinic would call to let me know how many eggs had fertilised, and two days later call again to let me know how many fertilised eggs were growing. The day before embryo-transfer day, the clinic would call to let me know how many fertilised eggs had developed into blastocyst embryos. Blastocyst embryos were what we wanted, as these embryos were five days old and ready to implant into the uterus wall.

And on embryo-transfer day the clinic would let me know how many they would transfer and how many they would freeze.

I would chat with my IVF friends about all of these numbers and they would say, *Oh, that is a good number. Wow, you got that many eggs retrieved,* and *Super wow, that many embryos now in the freezer.* It was like I felt proud of my numbers, especially when I compared them to others', but why? Oh, that's right, it was the years of conditioning from our society to compare ourselves to others.

And then there are the celebrities again; I can't help comparing myself to them for some reason. Maybe it is the glorified images we see of them in the magazines. Recently there has been a number of older celebrities who have given birth to babies, even twins. They have been in their late forties. It is great to hear them express their real story that they have used donor eggs, due to their own age and limited egg quality.

I have friends and family who have fallen pregnant easily, who have fallen pregnant unexpectedly, who have fallen pregnant without even trying. Who have fallen pregnant unexpectedly the first time and couldn't fall pregnant for a second when seriously trying. Who have had troubles falling pregnant the first time and suddenly fallen pregnant the second time. Also who were trying for a while, then sold up their house and left their jobs and went travelling around the country, then fell pregnant. Who have frozen their eggs as they haven't found their soulmate yet. Who have fallen pregnant with donor sperm. Who have had miscarriages early on and later in term. Who have had ectopic pregnancies and fallopian tubes removed and gone on to fall pregnant. Who have fallen pregnant with twins to discover one was ectopic and the other healthy, but ended up losing both while in emergency surgery. Who have had surgery to remove scar tissue and also their whole uterus.

These real-life examples only go to show how different everyone is. All our journeys are so contrasting. And even with the IVF journey, there are many variations between each couple. Some fall pregnant through IUI, some very lucky ones on their very first IVF cycle, and others on their tenth IVF cycle. As the famous quote says, life is a journey, not a destination.

When it comes to comparisonitis, become more self-aware and notice your triggers. Social media is a huge trigger for most people. How many times have you felt good and then started scrolling and suddenly felt bad?

Some things to consider are:

- *Scrolling: Be mindful about going onto social media. If you are feeling low, do not go online; it will trigger comparisons to others, especially a feeling of lack if you see pregnancy bellies and babies. Be more purposeful with your time on social media rather than aimlessly scrolling. Before you go online, list the things you want to look up and stick to them, this will bring you back in control rather than having your feed take you down a never-ending road. If a certain person or business is making you feel inferior, stop following them. I only follow positive people and have unfollowed many who do not ignite joy. Before you go online, ask yourself this simple question: Will this add meaning or value to my life? And if it won't, don't do it.*

- *Seeing filtered lives online: When people put carefully filtered images of themselves online, remember that this is only one very small part of their lives that they are choosing to put out there. You never really know what goes on behind closed doors.*

- *Focus on gratitude: When you feel triggered, stop and remind yourself of the items on your gratitude list – the one we discussed in Chapter 10. This will help you shift quickly out of comparison.*

- *Flip comparison around: Who do you follow on social media that you look up to? Flip your envy into something positive and follow inspiring people who are real and generous and making a difference in the world. Use this to fuel your own inner fire, pay it forward and inspire others.*

Instead of comparing yourself to others, change this around and compare yourself with you. How can you be a more loving and kinder person? What things can you do to improve your life? What can you learn from yesterday to be a better version of yourself today?

Choose love over fear and start within yourself. Are you doing that next round of IVF out of pure love for a baby or out of fear of being alone, or that your body clock is ticking, or that all your friends have babies so you should as well?

I definitely wanted a baby out of fear. I thought that because everyone else had a baby, we should too, and also I didn't want to be alone when I was older. However, now when I really sit with these thoughts—knowing that I have frozen embryos just sitting there—and ask myself if I still really want a baby out of pure love, the answer is not really. It would have to be a hands-down *Hell yes*, but it's just not there.

Sit with these feelings and go deeply within, as there you will find your answer.

If you catch yourself with negative self-talk—such as *Why is she pregnant with her third when I'm not even pregnant with my first?* or *Why does she fall pregnant so easily and it's taking so long for me?*—stop and recognise these thoughts as fear and comparison. Try to shift these negative thoughts and tell yourself a better story. Tell yourself that you are worthy of a baby, that you are worthy of being a mum, that your time will come. Have your very own power motto, this can be just a few words, but say it to yourself regularly during the day. It could be something like, *I am worthy of love and I am worthy of being a mother.* Say it whenever you are driving and stop at a traffic light, say it before you brush your teeth or after. This will help quickly redirect your thoughts to positivity.

When you are on the baby making train, remember that this is just a snapshot of your life right now. It is not the end of the movie that is your life. It might be where you are today, but things most likely will be different in the years to come. Focus on your mindset, your positive attitude, gratitude, and how you can make a difference in the world for the better.

# staying sane tips

1. *Everyone's baby journey is so different, just look around at your own family and friends and you will find that it wasn't smooth sailing for everyone.*

1. *Recognise if social media scrolling triggers your feelings of comparisonitis. If it does, start to be more aware of your social media usage.*

2. *Limit aimless scrolling on social media. Before you go online, make a list of what you want to look at and stick to it. And keep the timeframe short.*

3. *If you are already feeling down, do not go on social media. Only go online to directly look up people who inspire you.*

4. *Change up comparing yourself to others by comparing yourself to you. Bring the focus back to you and what you can improve within yourself.*

5. *Choose love over fear. Are you really doing that next IVF cycle out of pure love?*

6. *Take notice of any negative self-talk that's comparing yourself to others. Stop and redirect these thoughts into*

*positive self-talk. Tell yourself that your time will come to be a mother.*

7. *Remember that this won't last forever, it is just for now. You can take back your own power.*

8. *Book recommendation:* Comparisonitis *by Melissa Ambrosini. This book is a must for anyone trying to conceive.*

# 12

# More than just FOMO: deep fear

It seems that this little word, fear, can have such a big focus in our lives. Yes, there is FOMO, the fear of missing out when others are experiencing something exciting or interesting that you are not, often aroused by posts seen on social media. But there is also deep-down fear.

There is fear of being all alone, especially when you are old. Fear that you won't fall pregnant. Fear that you have left it too late. Fear that if you have children or grandchildren, they won't visit you when you are older and in a retirement village or nursing home.

I had all the fears, especially when it came to babies. Fear of miscarriage, fear of mid-term pregnancy loss, fear of stillbirth, fear of SIDS, fear of infancy sickness, fear of postnatal depression, fear of getting vaccinated or not, fear of driveway accidents or any random accident (such as a TV falling on the baby), fear of my child getting abducted walking to school or pinched from the front yard, fear of teenage car accidents, and fear of them getting stabbed or king hit while out on the town, let alone all the fears of a child getting into drugs and alcohol, and teen pregnancy. All these fears and I hadn't even fallen pregnant.

We really do live in a fear-based world. I also have so many other non-baby-related fears. I have worked in the travel industry booking flights for so many people, yet I have a fear of flying. I love take off and landing, but if there is the slightest bump when flying over the ocean, I'm hanging on for dear life—even though I know flying is much safer than driving in a car.

With fear, the logical brain goes out the window. I am fearful when any of my family is travelling long distances by car or planes. When my husband travels for work interstate or overseas, I track his plane on a flight-tracker website; I even keep the webpage open all day when I'm at work and keep looking at it. It's like a drug I have to keep having. Funnily enough, my older sister does the same with her grown-up children when they fly overseas. And even more funny is that my own mum gets anxious with us all-very-grown-up kids. Recently I travelled to Fiji on a girls trip and called my mum at the airport and she was like, 'I don't like when you kids fly out of the country,' and I'm the youngest and I'm forty!

I have this big fear that something bad will happen if I don't do things in a certain way. Yep, call this full-blown obsessive compulsive disorder (OCD). When I was growing up, I didn't know it had a name, I just thought I was weird. For me it is the repetition of things, that some objects need to be in the right place or that I need to do certain things in the right way and if I don't than something bad will happen My logical brain knows that this sounds totally crazy, but when you have had something like this since a child, it becomes your normal, like your own unique quirks.

One of my biggest fears is that I didn't fall pregnant because of my inner fear, anxiety, and OCD. In our doctors' eyes, everything was fine physically; my husband and all my tubes, eggs and age were all great, just a slight uterus issue. But nothing physically was stopping me from falling pregnant. Therefore, my mind wanders to the fear that it was because of my crazy anxious mind that I didn't fall pregnant and give my husband a child. That the universe is like, *Hell no, she already cray cray, don't give her a baby to screw up.*

How ironic that my fear is my fear. The anxiety is something that I wish I didn't have as I can feel very trapped sometimes; my outer self knows it's irrational, but my inner self thinks it's the norm. Argh, the lovely subconscious mind and its thoughts.

Another big fear that some of my IVF friends have is that they left it too late. And this fear mostly falls on women, as our reproductive body clock seems to flatline suddenly, before we even know it. There is no personalised strategic graph or Gantt chart PowerPoint presentation showing our decline in egg quality or likelihood of falling pregnant naturally and giving birth. However, these friends didn't meet their partners until later in life, as in their twenties they were travelling, working and partying. Then in your early thirties you focus on your career to save money to buy a house, and then it's a few years of working to pay off the top part of that house mortgage. Then you meet someone and date them for a few years and get married. And wow, you are pretty much forty before you even know it. But you don't look forty like our mothers and grandmothers did before us, as we know how to dress and do our makeup, have so many health and beauty products, and hair salons, and generally mix with a lot of different people of various ages and backgrounds, therefore we are more open to new ideas.

My baby fear now that I am forty is that I'm too old and no longer have the energy to have a pregnancy and newborn baby—getting up all hours of the night, and being glued to a baby all hours of the day. As I have been independent all my adult life, so to suddenly not have the freedom to go out whenever or wherever would be challenging.

Also there's fear of money, as raising kids is expensive. If we feel like we don't have enough money now, how on earth can we afford a child? Also, we would be financially responsible for the child from forty up until I'm sixty. And then I would want to retire, but probably wouldn't be able to afford to.

Another fear is that we would be the oldest parents at school drop off, how would we make friends with the other young parents? And OMG what would they think of us?

And then I have a fear that others will think I'm selfish because I haven't had children, that I was a 'childless by choice'!

And then a selfish fear I have is of losing my figure if I have a baby. I know this is so silly and very superficial as so many women have babies and healthy bodies. If I did put on weight, I think my self-esteem would really be affected. And I fear what others would think of me. Especially since I have been slim all my life and my older sisters are slim—they have both had kids and look terrific—I fear judgement that I was slack and couldn't lose the baby weight. For all the inner work I do on myself, it sounds so artificial to be worried about my appearance.

Another fear that pops up at random moments is the fear of deciding what to do with the embryos we have in the freezer. At this very moment the likelihood of us trying for a baby with these is pretty small. And now I have a fear about what to do with them. If we decide to not use them, do we get them destroyed (wow, so harsh sounding), or donate them? I have friends who have had their baby and are going through the process of donating their embryos to another lovely couple that they know. How cool is that? I kind of think I would like to donate them as we went through so much to get them, and they were retrieved at a time when we were so healthy, so I think they would be good quality. However, I would want to know if the embryos took and became babies. And then there is that fear of knowing you have a biological child out there—what do they look like, what is their personality? But the stupid fear is, *What if they want to meet us when they grow up and want to know why we donated them?* And another silly fear, *What if they randomly meet one of our relatives and they don't know it?*

With pregnancies, at an older age there is the fear of your child being born with Down syndrome. This is such a controversial one that I don't even know what I would do. I know that I would have my religious upbringing in my head that all life is precious and cannot be destroyed even when unborn. If I found out that our baby had Down syndrome and terminated the pregnancy, I would feel guilty for the rest of my life, I absolutely know that I would. I think I would have to go back to the old, scary church and do confession every Sunday. However, if we did go through with the pregnancy, it would change the rest of our lives—as any child does, of course, but it would be to a different level. And the selfish me doesn't know how I would cope. It is such a hard decision and I don't envy anyone who has had to go through this.

All throughout my life, I have pretty much worried about what other people think of me. Especially in my teenage years and twenties. Everything I did, I would be thinking of what others thought, and I would do things to make others approve of me or shy away from situations altogether. In my thirties that slowly went away and now I love who I am and know that others love me for me. Not because I am trying to be something different.

This fear of what other people think also applied to us not having a baby. What would they think of us if we had been married for five years and hadn't had a baby yet, or ten years, let alone fifteen years? And it's not like we were vocal and said right from the start that we were never wanting kids. Now I'm at a stage where I think that others will think that we are not having kids and I'm good with that. I also now just do what pleases me and makes my heart sing and it feels great.

Just as the lyrics to *Meant To Be* say, *If it's meant to be, it'll be, it'll be, Baby, just let it be.* We try to force so much in our lives, always hustling, chasing, pushing—many times in an effort to drown out or beat fear. We can live in either love or fear. However, fear can easily take over when we stop seeing love. Wouldn't it be amazing if we lived each day in a state of love and positivity?

Some small stepping stones you can take would be to bring in little bits of love and positivity each day. It might not be possible to overhaul absolutely everything at once but try to gradually notice any fearful thoughts and write them down. Or notice and rationally think about how they came to be. Once you dissect them, you will most likely see them differently and think how silly they were in the first place.

Worrying about the future doesn't get you anywhere, it just makes you more fearful. Dream up big goals instead and focus on pursuing them. What do you really want? What lights you up?

I know when I get fearful about the unknown future and all the bad things that could happen, I bring myself back to now and my goals. It absolutely works. Write down your goals and put up your vision board on the wall.

As we seem to be surrounded by fear, turn off the TV news channels, don't follow police updates on Facebook. Unsubscribe from news on your phone. We don't need to know this stuff. If something does happen to a loved one you will be notified. We don't need to bring the news of people getting stabbed and shot into our home, our sanctuary.

If you have a strong fear that if you don't have children, you will be all alone in old age, wouldn't it be even sadder if you did have children and they didn't come and visit you? There are no guarantees that by having children they will take care of you in old age, sad as that sounds.

Therefore, focus on your relationships with your family and friends and your interests. What lights you up? If you are worried about what other people will think of your passion project, just focus on how that passion project makes you feel. How it sparks something inside you. Do what feels good to you.

With the fear that you have left having babies too late, that your biological clock and egg quality diminished just when you were finally ready to have a baby, remember there is nothing that you can do to change the past. What has happened has happened. Stop dwelling on shoulda, wouldna, couldna. This might sound harsh, but it is true, you cannot change the past. You only did what you thought was the best thing at that time in your life. Yes, it can be unfair that the male reproductive clock does not tick as fast as the female one. However, no good comes from beating yourself up over it. You lived your earlier life in the moment and experienced things that you probably wouldn't have if you had had a baby in your early twenties.

Again, bring your focus back to now and your big goals and dreams. Not just goals of having a baby—your other passion project goals. Do you want to travel around a country in a campervan, learn to paint or walk a famous trail? Dream it and you will see it.

Another super helpful thing to get yourself out of Fear Town and into Self-Love Town is to read or listen to podcasts. I always have an amazing inspo book or two on the go. My bedside table usually has a pile of books on it as well as an e-reader. There is something magical about picking up or listening to an amazing book, or when you are driving or out walking and listening to a great positivity-infused podcast. If you only pick up on one little hint or takeaway, this can help with fear so much.

# staying sane tips

1.  *Notice any fearful thoughts you have and write them down. By writing them down, you are giving them less power and looking at them in a different light, which will help you change that fearful thought or remove it altogether.*

2.  *Focus on your big goals and dreams. Put together a vision board by cutting out pictures of things, places and people you want in your life that make you happy. And if worries come up about the scary unknown future, direct your focus to your vision board and big goals instead.*

3.  *Turn off the news TV channels and news email subscriptions, unfollow police Facebook pages, etc. There is no good in bringing these fearful events into your home sanctuary.*

4.  *Focus on what lights you up inside, what things make your inner self jump for joy. Pursue your passion projects as this will make your heart sing.*

5.  *If you fear that you have left starting a family too late, stop beating yourself up. There are many people who have started a family later in life and it can happen. No good will come from you beating yourself up about it.*

6. *Get yourself into anything positive: books, audiobooks, blogs, podcasts. These good vibes will get you out of a funk and into a clear headspace instantly.*

# 13

# Your cheer squad and your partner in crime

Can I get a B, A, B, Y, gooooooo baby!

For many of our big life events, and life in general, we have our cheer squad, our support group, family, friends, gang, crew, mates, BFFs, etc. But what happens when you are experiencing something that is usually deemed a private matter ... conceiving, having sex, trying to make a baby? When you are longing for that day when you can surprise your cheer squad with your pregnancy news? What happens when that "surprise" never comes and one of your hardest journeys is just about to begin and you feel all alone?

This journey through infertility treatment will require your best cheer squad ever. But who can you trust to cheer you on during this very personal journey? Who is going to hold your hand when you can't see out of the dark tunnel? And has anyone ever been through this before you who can offer their advice?

I don't think I could even count up how many hours I have spent talking to my cheer squad about babies, or my lack of— conversations and D & Ms about my baby-making train ride, or more like train wreck, with my cheer squad over coffee, long lunches, phone calls, emails, text messages, Zoom calls to Ireland, road trips, flights and overseas holidays. We have talked it raw and to the bone.

## THE FAM BAM CHEER SQUAD

But it wasn't always so easy. When I first started trying for a baby, only a couple of people knew, as they had just had babies and I would listen so intently to their stories of pregnancy, birth and breastfeeding like I was educating myself for future reference when my time came. However, it never came. I eventually told my sisters and my mum, but that was after a good few years of trying the natural way, and when I opened up to them, it was so freeing, like a pressure had been lifted. I had been conditioned to think the perfect story was to find a guy, settle down, get married and start a family. A career and travel were just on the side. As mentioned, when I was growing up, I would always play with dolls and Barbies, and I never played with briefcases or model planes. So when I opened up just a little with my fam bam, that expectation I had put on myself to be perfect was slightly released.

## MY BFFS

I opened up to a few of my BFFs, as we naturally had organic conversations where we didn't need to pretend we were perfect. We would go back and forth about all the new things I could try: supplements, herbal teas, natural remedies, books to read ... all the things. It was like a coaching session before a big game. And we'd also discuss all the fears: fear of failure, fear of money, fear of life balance. Just knowing I had my besties on speed dial was a huge comfort. Their support to me was invaluable and I can never thank them enough for all their positive energy and encouragement.

## MY FELLOW IVF-ERS

A game changer for me on this crazy train ride was when I dragged my depressed butt off the couch and got myself to an IVF support group for a coffee and chat. As no one in my circle of friends and family had gone through infertility, finding my fellow IVF-ers was a complete turning point. I no longer felt like I was the only one going through this journey, I had buddies to share my struggles with who had also gone through these same struggles. Once I opened this gate, my world also opened up. It was just so freeing to have my inner perfectionism exposed.

My cheer squad really became essential when I started doing IVF, as it is a whole different ball game to just trying to fall pregnant naturally. With all the planning and scheduling that goes into an IVF cycle, my cheer squad were interested in what stage I was at and we would exchange suggestions. I cannot stress how freeing it was to open up to like-minded people who were there to help me and I felt more useful in that I could reciprocate this as well.

## MY EXPERTS DREAM TEAM

Just like Beyoncé has her dream team ready her for a concert

... I had my dream team ready me for my baby. This was my fertility expert dream team that I was seeing for treatments. My naturopaths, acupuncturists, kinesiologists and Chinese medicine practitioners.

When you see your dream team weekly or fortnightly during an IUI or IVF cycle, they really do become a huge support, but their support is more of a practical look at what new things can be done to increase your odds of falling pregnant. I always felt so amazing after I would see my dream team as I didn't feel so isolated and could get their advice on the little things going through my head, such as, *I was thinking of going camping after the embryo transfer, is this ok?* or *I have my softball grand final game coming up, should I run?* Even talking on Zoom to my naturopath was amazing.

Having your expert dream team around you really helps get you out of your own head and excites you for the possibility of your future baby.

## MY FUN SQUAD

So I was very lucky to have my fam bam, besties, fellow IVF-ers and expert dream team around me, but what I also discovered after going through infertility for a while was that I needed my "let's get messy" fun friends.

With living in a suburb that is very oriented to young families and working in a big office where there was always a heap of girls pregnant, discovering my fun friends was invaluable to finding myself and all the things that I love doing. I played softball on weekends with a mixed bunch of women and it was great for socialising, laughing, and getting fresh air and exercise, and I didn't feel anyone's eyes on me with the expectation of babies.

My newly discovered fun friends didn't have kids and we would go out in the city and dance like no one was watching. Sometimes a girl has just gotta have a good dance and get messy!

Ok so there were a few hangovers the following day, but during the dance party times I discovered that there were happy couples out there who didn't have kids and had full, purposeful lives! Wow, this was seriously a concept that I had never thought of before ... could people lead purposeful lives without having kids? I observed first hand that yes, they could and actually did.

Also, we were lucky that we could go out on a whim without having to get a babysitter and be home by a certain time, or fall asleep at 9.00 pm due to child exhaustion. And we could go travelling without having to plan it around school holidays. It was kind of freeing and turned into a new chapter for my husband and me.

A bunch of my fun friends will read this book who never knew that we went through IVF for years. But that is ok, as I needed them to be my fun friends, my adventure friends and my dance buddies.

I absolutely love, cherish and appreciate all of my cheer squads, I definitely could not have made it through infertility without them. However, sometimes I just really needed to do tequila shots and dance without thinking about infertility treatments.

## YOUR PARTNER IN CRIME

You were so excited on your wedding day to get married to your spouse, you even saved the top tier of your wedding cake to freeze and bring out on the day of your firstborn's christening. And when you were searching for your new family home together, a requirement was that it had to have lots of spare bedrooms and a big backyard to fill with kids, and also a parent's retreat where you could escape with your other half. However, how do you feel when it is still just the two of you sitting at the big dining table after a few years of trying to fill your family home with kids' laughter?

How does your marriage survive infertility: the uncertainty, expenses, emotional ups and downs, and the scheduled everything, from medical appointments to sex. And for your husband who desperately wants that baby as well, but feels like he is helpless as you are the one having all the medical procedures, as he can't take the blood tests or hormone injections, or have the egg retrieval procedures, this part is all one sided. How does your once carefree, fun and lighthearted relationship go when things get tough—when you are both not getting what you want, and that is to be parents. And if your partner was infertile, would you stay together if it meant that you would not become a parent?

Research shows that infertility can put a strain on a marriage, especially long-term failed fertility treatments. Also, another pressure within a marriage is the decision of continuing on with treatments, or not—what if one partner wants to continue on and the other doesn't? Who gets to decide, and at what cost?

So yes, in good Catholic style we had kept the top tier of our wedding cake and put it in the freezer. However, unlike my sisters, it didn't come out a year or two after our wedding at our first baby's christening ... it ended up staying in that freezer for years. When we did defrost it, it didn't look too good as the white icing had gone a yellowish colour and I don't remember it tasting particularly good.

So when we bought our house, it had a few spare bedrooms and a separate master bedroom with an ensuite at the other end of the house, which is exactly what I had wanted, kind of like the parents retreat. It was a brand-new home in a brand-new suburb that was completely geared towards young families. At times when I was home alone, cleaning the house, I would excitedly walk into the spare bedroom that I thought was going to be our nursery and imagine what curtains I would put up and where I would put the cot and change table. Other times I would walk past that room and glance in and feel all alone, empty.

However, I never shared these thoughts and feelings with my amazing husband. But why shouldn't I have? We were on this journey together, equal parts in a journey to parenthood.

Growing up, although my family went to church every Sunday, we never said that we loved each other out loud. It was like it was a given, so we didn't need to say it. However, when I meet my hubby's family, they were very vocal with their affection. But still, talking about my feelings never came naturally to me. Therefore, in the early years of trying to fall pregnant, I mostly kept my feelings in, only a rare escape here and there. Each month when I would find out that I wasn't pregnant, I just carried on, I never even told my husband. I think I didn't want to get my hopes up, so I thought if I was pregnant it would be a big surprise and then I would tell him and we'd be so happy in that moment together. I was good at sharing my happy and excited feelings but not so good at sharing my sadness as I didn't want to make him sad as well. I felt like I was letting him down.

When our very first IVF embryo transfer didn't work—and I had so thought that it would as we had put so much into it physically, emotionally and mentally—I was devastated. I cried in the dark in our bedroom, lying on the bed, curled up in the fetal position alone. My husband was home but I didn't want him to see me because I didn't want to make him sad. But he had an equal part in the journey, so why didn't I let him in? I think I didn't because I'm usually a person that just gets straight back up when I get knocked down—I brush myself off and move forward. Being stuck in this downer was strange ground for me and I didn't know how to deal with it, so I felt I needed to deal alone. However, my husband found me crying in the bedroom and held me tight and said that I was never to cry alone in the dark again. That we were in this together in every way, the good and bad.

As I sit here now, writing these words in the very same bedroom with my coffee in hand, it brings tears to my eyes. I have nearly finished writing my story in this book and none of my previous words about our baby-making train ride have brought tears to my eyes, but when I write about my husband telling me to never cry in the dark again, I'm instantly in tears. Loving tears of him being my rock and my amazing partner in crime.

He is the best thing about my life. He has always been so good with words and expressing himself; when we were first dating, he would write me beautiful words in notes and cards, which I still have today. He has encouraged me to open up about the good and the bad, and shown me that it doesn't always have to be roses, it can be darkness as well. And that is what a true partnership is.

I think that sometimes, especially as women, we want to solve others' problems, make everyone else feel better, encourage others to get back up and get back out there. We like to soothe and soften others in their challenging situations. We deflect so much of the inward attention on ourselves and push it back to others because doing the inner work on ourselves can at times be painful. We don't feel worthy of receiving help as we have grown up in an environment where women nurture everyone else but themselves. And we keep our struggles of infertility a secret because we don't want to burden others or feel ashamed that we can't conceive a child.

There are many professions out there where the star person appears as themselves. Just look at a professional tennis player, they go out on the court and play the game by themselves. Even when they take a break on the sideline, they look all alone. And they do the press tours and interviews on their own as well. However, that tennis player has their team sitting in the player box cheering them on: their coach, trainer, doctor, physiotherapist, friends and family. They travel together, train together, discuss game plans together, eat and rest together. This tennis player would never be able to get to their number-one world ranking without their very own cheer squad.

And if someone is unfortunately diagnosed with a disease, that person will be offered a full list of people to see who can assist them medically and emotionally. Friends, family and colleagues will rally around them to cheer them on. It is human nature to want to assist someone who is struggling with something.

So going through infertility and IVF shouldn't be any different. Your closest will want to help you and cheer you on. So let them in, open up and accept the warming feeling of comfort from people who truly want to help you. You don't need to open up to everyone all at once or post it on social media if that makes you feel exposed, but gradually open up to your nearest and dearest. And do this with the intention of simply releasing your inner emotional turmoil, and with no expectation of others fixing you.

When you truly open up to your cheer squad and partner in crime, you will instantly feel the weight of the world lifted off your shoulders. And when you are starting a new round of IVF, that feeling of having one less thing weighing you down is so important. Letting your cheer squad in on what is happening will help you through the needles, medical procedures and two-week wait—especially so if it is a negative result. They won't be able to fix your problem, but they will help strengthen your mindset, which is the core of your being.

Don't cry alone. If a negative pregnancy test makes you hit rock bottom, remember that you are not in this alone, your partner is equal on your journey to parenthood. Open up and let them in; open communication will bring you closer together. Talk about what you are going through, instead of just putting on Netflix and masking the pain. Feeling your emotions now will enable you to release them and help you both get back up and move forward.

Also, don't beat yourself up if you just want to let your hair down and party where there is no talk of doctors, injections or fertility treatments. Sometimes you can get so fixated on getting that baby that you forget who you were before IVF, and also your marriage before infertility. Remember that you can still want a baby and want to be a parent with your spouse while also wanting to just let loose and have some good ol' fashioned fun. And you know what, if you wake up with a headache the next morning from too much dancing the night before, that is ok. You had a fun time with your partner and friends, you laughed, you danced and it felt good. Remember to do things that make you feel good.

With infertility, it can be a challenge to do what Oprah says and live in the moment, as so much of IVF is forward planning. However, it is important to take a break from that to recharge, physically and mentally. And to share fun experiences with your cheer squad and partner, where there is no talk of infertility. Give yourself time to reconnect with yourself.

# staying sane tips

1. *It is ok to do the inner work on yourself. Yes, it might bring up painful emotions and shame that you can't conceive a child, but going within and releasing any held emotions will greatly help you move forward in life with whatever happens.*

1. *Remember, even professionals have a team around them to cheer them on and direct them on their next step, so it is ok for you to have your cheer squad as well.*

2. *Let your cheer squad and partner in on any tightly held emotions with the intention of getting them off your chest. This will help you release the emotions and feel lighter.*

3. *Meditate using one simple word: release. Sit quietly and close your eyes and repeat the word with every breath. This one word has so many meanings and is very powerful.*

4. *Cry and let your emotions out with your partner, as it will strengthen your relationship and bring you closer together on this journey.*

5. *Remember who you were before IVF and your marriage before infertility, go out and have some fun and live in the moment.*

# My final words and thoughts (for now)

For many years I was in a haze, thinking that my life would "start" when I fell pregnant and had a baby. I feared the times when my mind wasn't occupied at work or busily doing "things" as that meant I had free time to think and I would always be thinking about my lack of a baby, that something was missing in my life … that I wasn't whole.

But now that I'm on the other side of my *trying to have a baby* years, babies don't even come into my mind. And if they do, it is with a completely different feeling … kind of like I'm happy to not have had a baby. Which is SO strange, because I tried to have a baby for SO long. And I still have frozen embryos, so it's a really bizarre feeling to not want to use them anymore.

I have this excited feeling for all the new adventures life has to offer. I now see so many possibilities for all the things I can do, and I have the freedom to do them without having to think of how it might impact my child.

When I was in those trying years, I never once thought that I could feel whole without becoming a parent. And now I know that this is my purpose: to help people who have gone through failed infertility find themselves again, without feeling shame or that they are lacking something, and to help them embrace all their future possibilities with excitement.

Isn't it ironic how my purpose has turned out to be the gift underneath my experiences? And today it fuels me by serving my growth. Problems are what sculpt our soul, or in other words, the shit that you have gone through can ultimately lead you to a great place ... the silver linings. Finding your life purpose is really about inner growth from whatever experiences have challenged you to rise above and move forward with excitement. And I can vouch by saying that shit feels good!

My mission now is to start a global movement. What is the name for the group of people who wanted children but couldn't have them, and not for lack of trying? And when people ask you if you have children, you could just say this phrase and they would instantly understand ... with no judgement or further interrogation. That you are not childless by choice, you really wanted children but it didn't happen for you.

Instead of #mumlife, I'm starting a global movement called #embraceotherhood. To embrace otherhood is to know that you did all you could to have children and you know that being a parent would not singly define who you truly are, that you are whole and complete just as you are.

I want to help women release the shame around not becoming a mother and through connection I want to inspire them to feel excitement in living their best new life by embracing otherhood. No more suffering in silence or dealing with infertility trauma alone; by embracing otherhood we collectively seek transformation and new meaning.

I hope that you see the end of this book as the beginning of your new epic life in whatever form that may be for you.

I appreciate you for reading this book and I hope that it helps even just a little on your unique journey.

If you feel called to, please pay it forward by buying a copy and giving it to anyone you know who is experiencing infertility. Infertility can be such a silent pain, therefore by sharing this book you are personally contributing to the global movement by bringing more awareness to people who wanted children but couldn't have them and not for lack of trying. #embraceotherhood.

Please reach out to me personally at my email address below and share your unique story, as I would genuinely love to connect with you and hear your story.

If you wish to connect with a like-minded tribe, please go to my website or socials:

- *Website: www.embraceotherhood.com*
- *Email: hello@embraceotherhood.com*
- *Instagram: @embraceotherhood @bern_andrews*

I see you and I hear you, and please know that you are not alone. Remember, you are whole just as you are!

Take care,
Bernadette

# Acknowledgements

Writing this book came to me as a crazy idea when I was having a coffee with my fertility bestie Charlene. We were talking about all the people we'd met on our journey, all the tips we'd shared and all the crazy shit we'd done to try to fall pregnant. I'm sure that many a girlfriend group has had similar conversations, but when I got home from that coffee I did something about it … I got on my laptop and just started typing up bullet point notes.

At first it was coming from a place of frustration towards the people who had no idea, the work lunch room crowd who would say, *Oops, I just accidentally fell pregnant.* Then the typing started to change as I considered my future self; if I lost my memory in old age, I would have documented all the things I had done to have a baby and know that I had given it a good crack.

In the months following, I would add to my bullet points when I remembered other things or funny stories of my baby-making train ride. And on the brink of turning forty, I had this strong desire to join the bullet points together into a book.

However, self-doubt crept in as it usually does, all the usual questions such as *Who am I to write a book? You're not smart enough to write a book. You have started so many other things in the past and not finished them, what makes this different?* These questions prompted me to seek a coach, someone who could push me in the right direction and hold me accountable to actually write and finish this book.

And who would have thought that when I googled business coaches a fellow country girl from the neighbouring town to mine during my primary school years would pop up on my screen? Lizzie Moult, thank you so much for guiding me during the writing of this book; you helped me open up on the page and through my words. You kept me accountable each step of the way, and guided me back on track when I was getting derailed by life. And you helped me believe that this book is meant to be shared so that the women suffering in silence know they aren't alone. Thank you so much for your coaching and friendship.

To Natasha at the kind press, thank you for helping me publish this book. I have never written a book before or published anything, and your guidance has been amazing. I had this positive feeling when I submitted my book to you and when I was sitting on a beach at Moreton Island, reading your email that you'd like to publish my book, the good vibes were flowing. And your encouraging words in that email saying that there needs to be a book like this in the world has kept me going with the process, when that little self-doubt has crept in.

Thank you so much to my wonderful family, all of you, as I have my Murray Clan and crazy in-law fam bam, you are the best. Especially to my sisters, Regina and Lucinda, it is so nice to have close sisters and I'm grateful just knowing you are there for me in whatever I do.

Thank you to my besties who literally helped me stay sane on this crazy train. To Jade, I have had the pleasure of you being in my life since we were eighteen years old and flatmates. Jade, along with her hubby, Jason, introduced me to my husband, Quentin, all those years ago in November of 1996. Thank you for all your time, all the convos, all the coffees, brekkies, lunches, dinners, movies, walks, car rides, holidays, op shop visits and Zumba classes and all the phone calls, messages, emails, etc. I really value your true friendship. And you're also my photographer for this book and my website … thank you again!

To Sokar, who is my "anything goes" let's-do-a-white-Christmas bestie, thank you for your encouragement during the writing of this book. You were the first person other than my coach to read the first draft. Thank you for your advice in letting me know that this book needs to be published.

To my beautiful bestie Serena, thank you for your belief in me. I felt how proud you were of me in writing this book. You telling me of all the people who would really benefit from reading it has kept me going and helped me to finish and publish it.

And to all my fun-time besties, Kate (aka Keith, lol), Karen M, Lena, Lisa, Mel, Donna, Karen D, Charlene, Bronwyn, Martine, Billie, Christine, Dinelle, Naomi, Sam and Cat, just having fun with you all is the best thing. Life is about laughter and play even when we are big kids … oh and lots of wine, margaritas and dancing too.

And to the very best person in my life, my most favourite human in the world, my husband, Quentin: I'm so grateful that I get to share this crazy ride with you. We have shared so much on this journey and you only ever encouraged me, and funny how after surviving this crazy ride together we didn't need children to complete us as we are pretty special just as we are. Thanks, Babes, and I love you so much!

To my readers, I got out of my comfort zone and wrote this book with the hope that it would help you—even if just a little—to know that you are not alone and that your life is full of meaning and purpose.

With gratitude,
Bernadette xo

# About the author

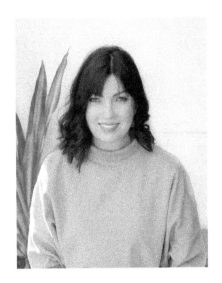

*Bernadette Andrews*

For sixteen years, Bernadette Andrews has been on and off the baby making train in the hopes of falling pregnant. She has done it all, from IVF and Chinese medicine to naturopathy, acupuncture, hypnotherapy, kinesiology and strict fertility food plans—all while maintaining her humorous and positive vibe.

In sharing her story, Bernadette hopes to help others experiencing infertility know they're not alone, and that you can live a full, purposeful and rewarding life whether you join the mothers club or not.